TWELVE KEY STRATEGIES
TO IMPROVE CASH FLOW
IN MEDICAL GROUPS

2nd edition

By
DAVID H. ZIMMERMAN

Center for Research in Ambulatory Health Care Administration
Research Arm of the Medical Group Management Association
Englewood, Colorado
July 1992

To my father, Eliot "Zim" Zimmerman, who has always supported and encouraged all of my accomplishments and who has been a great example to his children.

TABLE OF CONTENTS

PAGE

List of Figures IX

Foreword to Second Edition x

Foreword to First Edition xi

Preface xii

Letter from the Sponsor xiii

About the Center for Research in Ambulatory
Health Care Administration and the Medical
Group Management Association xiv

About the Author xv

INTRODUCTION 1

KEY STRATEGY 1 3

DEVELOP CONTROL PRIOR TO SERVICE
Obtaining Accurate Information
Advantages of Preregistration for a Group Practice
Advantages of Preregistration for Patients
Tips for Developing a Preregistration System
Scheduling and Business Office Liaison
Staff Training
Financial Responsibility
Ineffective Preregistration

KEY STRATEGY 2 9

SAFEGUARD CONTROL AT TIME OF SERVICE
Reduce the Surprise
The After-Service Interview
Sensing Problems Early
A Last-Chance Situation
Records Maintenance

KEY STRATEGY 3 13

NEUTRALIZE SMALL BALANCE ACCOUNTS
Examination of Present Systems
Different Management Techniques
Practical Policies
Updated and Specific Procedures
Tips for Collecting at Time of Service
A Unique Billing and Follow-up System

KEY STRATEGY 4 21
   IMPROVE STAFF ABILITY TO COLLECT
         Underqualified Collectors
         Underpaid Collectors
         Not Enough Collectors
         Auditing Collector Effectiveness
         Developing Good Collectors
         Building a Game Plan
         Questioning Techniques
         The Lombardi Rules

KEY STRATEGY 5 35
   CONCENTRATE COLLECTION EFFORTS ON INSURANCE
         Before and After
         Electronic Claims Processing
         Billing Control Reports
         Effective Follow-up Policy
         Preparation and Contact
         Visits to Insurance Companies
         Getting Others Involved
         Managed Care Contracts

KEY STRATEGY 6 43
   REDUCE SELF-PAY CONTRACTS
         Major Credit Cards
         Medical Credit Cards
         Bank Financing
         Payment Monitoring Programs

KEY STRATEGY 7 47
   DESIGN FORM LETTERS THAT WORK
         Why Patients Do Not Pay
         Collection Letters
         Insurance Follow-up Letters
         Collection Notices and Statements

KEY STRATEGY 8 59
   EXPAND DATA PROCESSING PAYOFF
         Guidelines for Management
         Accuracy of Aged Trial Balance
         Exception Reporting
         Effective Use of Statements

KEY STRATEGY 9 69

ANALYZE TO GET THE "BIGGEST BANG FOR THE BUCK"

Zeroing in on Major Problems

Payment History Analysis

Developing Goals from Analysis

Third-Party and Debtor Profile Analyses

Determining Individual Analytical Needs

KEY STRATEGY 10 75

BUILD GOOD PUBLIC RELATIONS

The Customers

The Manager

Collection Policy, Procedures, and Practices

Collection Notices and Letters

Scoring Public Relations Points

The Business Office

A Public Relations Training Program

Fielding Complaints

Answering Letters of Complaint

Good Service Makes Dollars and Sense

The Fair Debt Collection Practices Act

KEY STRATEGY 11 87

SET GOALS FOR DIRECTION, MOTIVATION, AND RESULTS

Goal Setting

Think Success

Managing Change

Motivation and Success

Management by Objectives

Setting Goals with Staff

Job Enrichment in Practice

KEY STRATEGY 12 105

MAXIMIZE COLLECTION AGENCY RECOVERY

Use of Outside Agencies

Selection Criteria

Commissions and Recovery Rate

Regular Listings and Cancellation of Accounts

Evaluation Criteria

Investigating Other Agencies

Attorneys for Collection

Importance of Analysis

Considering an In-House Agency

Going into Action

Opening to Other Clients

An Answer, a Challenge, and a Risk

APPENDIX A. WORKSHEETS 119

BIBLIOGRAPHY 139

LIST OF FIGURES

1-1	Sample Payment Agreements	7
3-1	Billing Cycles	17
3-2	A Total Collection System	18
4-1	Collector Review Form	25
4-2	Motivator Topics for Collecting	30
5-1	Proven Follow-up Techniques by Major Financial Class	38
7-1	Sample Collection Letters	49
7-2	Sample Insurance Follow-up Letters	53
7-3	Sample Statement Cycles	56
8-1	Collector Performance Report	63
8-2	Report Comparing Collections to Goal	64
8-3	Collection Agency Performance Report	65
9-1	Flowchart of Problem Identification	70
9-2	Payment History of Insurance Companies with More than One Occasion	72
9-3	Payment History Analysis per Patient	72
9-4	History Analysis of Write-Offs to Agencies	73
10-1	Collection Code of Ethics	77
10-2	Patient Complaint Form	80
10-3	Public Relations Problems and Solutions	83
11-1	Sequence of Actions for Management by Objectives	92
11-2	Sample Key Result Areas and Performance Indicators	95
11-3	Sample Completed Monthly Goal Status Report	96
11-4	Sample Completed Annual Action Plan	97
11-5	Sample Collection Strategy	101
11-6	Approaches to Job Enrichment	103
12-1	Comparison of Two Collection Agencies	109
12-2	Steps to Setting Up an In House Collection Agency	117

FOREWORD TO SECOND EDITION

As interest has intensified to limit fee increases and control the cost of physician services, there has been increasing pressure to improve the cash management of medical group practice through collection improvement. Addressing the management challenges involved, the Center for Research in Ambulatory Health Care Administration (CRAHCA) initiated a project in 1984 to define the key points involved in effective cash flow management. The first edition of this publication was developed from the idea that group practices must stabilize their cash flow through well managed collection procedures. This goal has increased in importance as the collections management process has become more complex through the increase in managed care and other contractual discount arrangements.

In 1985, CRAHCA published the first edition of *Twelve Key Strategies to Improve Cash Flow for Medical Groups* by David H. Zimmerman of Milwaukee, Wisconsin. In multiple printings, 3,000 copies of the first edition have been used to enhance cash flow management in medical group practice. We are indebted to Mr. Zimmerman for not only have authored the first edition, but in agreeing to update the text to address current collection management issues, with specific attention devoted to electronic billing, insurance collection management, and HMO/PPO contractual payments. In creating the second edition, the author has developed some additional worksheets and all of the worksheets have been placed in one section to facilitate reproduction.

CRAHCA would like to acknowledge the continued support of CyCare Systems, Incorporated of Phoenix, Arizona and Dubuque, Iowa for its funding of both the first and second editions and continued interest in fulfilling the needs of medical group management. Appreciation is extended to the people who contributed to the updating of the first edition. In addition to the author who made substantial changes to several chapters, Janice Pramik provided comprehensive editorial support and insured consistency throughout the publication. Christopher J. Baca, Administrator, Department of Surgery, University of Texas Medical Branch at Galveston, Galveston, Texas, and Margaret L. Stone, Administrator, Toledo Clinic and Outpatient Surgery Center, Toledo, Ohio, shared their working knowledge in their capacities as reviewers of this second edition.

Margaret L. Stone also participated in the development of the first edition by contributing her expertise to the author through the interview process and as a reviewer of the first edition.

A final and important acknowledgement is given to the Center for Research in Ambulatory Health Care Administration staff whose editing, word processing, project management and supervision of the printing were essential to completing the task of producing this publication. Thank you, David N. Gans, Senior Project Director and Lisa E. Pieper, Administrative Assistant. Barbara Hamilton, Director of the MGMA Library Resource Center updated the comprehensive bibliography.

Englewood, Colorado
June 1992

Steven S. Lazarus, PhD
Associate Executive Director
Center for Research in
Ambulatory Health Care
Administration

FOREWORD TO FIRST EDITION

As public interest in medical costs and services intensifies, medical institutions are charged to control rates and, at the same time, to extend hours of operation and include a wider variety of services. Recognizing the implications of these challenges, the Center for Research in Ambulatory Health Care Administration (Center for Research) initiated this project to define key points involved in effective cash flow management. This publication was developed from the idea that if group practices are to become better equipped to expand their services, they must first stabilize their cash flow, and because patient accounts represent a major resource in a cash flow scheme, establishing a systematic collection procedure to cover all aspects of patient accounts is essential.

As publisher of *Twelve Key Strategies to Improve Cash Flow in Medical Groups*, the Center for Research would like to thank those who contributed to this work, particularly the author, David H. Zimmerman, Milwaukee, Wisconsin, whose dedication and expertise made this book a reality, and CyCare Systems, Incorporated, of Dubuque, Iowa, for its funding and interest in fulfilling the needs of the medical community.

Special appreciation is extended to the people who contributed to the content through interviews with the author. Their sharing of their knowledge and experiences significantly added to the ideas contained in the body of this work. They are: Rodney K. Amundson*, Assistant Administrator, Wilkinson Clinic, SC, Oconomowoc, Wisconsin; Robert L. Downs, FACMGA*, Executive Director, Midelfort Clinic, Limited, Eau Claire, Wisconsin; Jim H. Houtz, President*, CyCare Systems, Incorporated, Dubuque, Iowa; Frances Weier, Administrator, Doctors Clinic, Limited, Two Rivers, Wisconsin; Joe Hancock, Product Analyst, CyCare Systems, Incorporated, Dubuque, Iowa; Peg L. Stone*, Senior Vice President, Nicolet Clinic, SC, Neenah, Wisconsin; and Joseph J. Dillenberg*, Administrator, Willmar Medical Center, Willmar, Minnesota.

*Also, thank you to the reviewers of the text; with their input the completeness of this publication was assured.

A final acknowledgement to the Center for Research staff whose editing, word processing, and supervision of typesetting and printing helped finalize the manuscript for publication. Thank you, Ralph R. Gayner, Project Director; Mary Jo Ross, Administrative Assistant; Ann Madden, Secretary; and Pat Doty, Secretary.

Denver, Colorado
October 1985
Mary Alice Krill, PhD
Administrative Director
and Director of Research
Center for Research
in Ambulatory Health
Care Administration

PREFACE

The challenge of keeping accounts receivables in check while containing costs and maintaining collection totals faces group administrators and accounts receivable managers every day. The twelve sections of this book serve as an outline of key areas involved in this challenge. Though there may be other areas, we feel these are the most pertinent to medical group collection and cash flow today.

In compiling this book, we have included both the specifics of group collection systems and the less defined human element. The mix of these two major components is sometimes referred to as the "art and science" of managing receivables. The content also centers on public relations concerns encountered when dealing with patients, as well as on the internal structure of a group's collection staff. As such, job enrichment is highlighted within these twelve strategies.

The step-by-step structure of the book lends itself to the sequence involved in medical group collection and cash flow. The nature of collecting from insurance companies, and self-pay and small balance accounts, among other categories, is approached through various information-gathering techniques, analysis of collection totals and collector data, staff training and management, data processing reporting, and goal setting. Public relations and job enrichment are covered as major factors affecting the collection efforts and cash flow of medical groups.

Sections of this publication are designed in a workbook fashion. As you review the text, you will note the narrative is supported by illustrations and examples; sample worksheets and output reports are included. Material for this book was gathered during my years of experience as a health care accounts receivable manager and consultant. We hope you will find the information and methods contained in these twelve key areas helpful in your efforts to achieve improved collection and cash flow for your medical group.

David H. Zimmerman
President
David H. Zimmerman & Associates
Milwaukee, Wisconsin
June 1992

LETTER FROM THE SPONSOR

Dear Reader,

In 1984, CyCare Systems, Incorporated, was contacted by the Center for Research in Ambulatory Health Care Administration, regarding the possibility of its funding the development of a group practice collection manual. We agreed to assist the Center for Research and felt the finished product would be extremely helpful to medical group practices.

CyCare Systems, Incorporated was pleased to be able to continue its funding support for this project with a grant to partially offset the expenses incurred in publishing the second edition as part of our continuing commitment to enhance collections management

This second edition covers additional topics, electronic billing, insurance collection, and HMO/PPO payment; all of which have receive increased attention.

The increasing competition among healthcare delivery systems is characterized by a shift from traditional financial mechanisms to prepaid plans. Even so, the collection function is still an important part of the management of patient accounts and cash flow. In addition, the ever increasing pressures on providers to moderate healthcare costs will demand greater cost containment efforts from all of us.

We feel confident this second edition of *Twelve Key Strategies to Improve Cash Flow in Medical Groups* will make a significant contribution to your efforts.

Sincerely,

Jim H. Houtz
President
CyCare Systems, Incorporated
Scottsdale, Arizona
June 1992

ABOUT THE CENTER FOR RESEARCH IN AMBULATORY HEALTH CARE ADMINISTRATION AND THE MEDICAL GROUP MANAGEMENT ASSOCIATION

The Center for Research in Ambulatory Health Care Administration (CRAHCA), established in 1973, is a section 501(c)(3) tax-exempt charitable organization as defined by the Internal Revenue Code. The purpose of CRAHCA is to improve ambulatory health care in general and group practice in particular through better administration. Its work focuses on new and innovative publications; education, research, and data services; and demonstration programs. The Center for Research in Ambulatory Health Care Administration is the research arm of the Medical Group Management Association (MGMA).

Founded in 1926, the Medical Group Management Association is the oldest and largest membership organization representing group practice administration. MGMA serves its individual and organizational members and their patients, and promotes the group practice of medicine as an effective and efficient form of health care delivery. MGMA is comprised of more than 12,000 individual and 5,000 medical group practice members. More than 104,000 physicians practice in MGMA member groups.

ABOUT THE AUTHOR

David H. Zimmerman has acquired significant expertise through his work in health care accounts receivable consultation, organizational analysis, managerial auditing, educational development, and supervisory training.

Zimmerman received his Bachelor of Science degree from the University of Wisconsin. He has held a variety of health care financial management positions including vice president of a hospital-owned collection agency, director of patient business services, business manager, and patient accounts manager in a large hospital. Prior to becoming a consultant, Zimmerman served as director of education services for the Healthcare Financial Management Association where his responsibilities included directing national educational programs and services. He is an experienced seminar leader on health care topics and developer of in-house training courses for hospitals and other health care organizations.

The author has proven himself a manager of problems and challenges in health care accounts receivable management. Among other accomplishments, Zimmerman successfully dealt with and maintained an outstanding days revenue average of under 45 days over a ten-year period in the same metropolitan hospital. He has received the Wisconsin Hospital Manager of the Year Award from the Associated Hospital Services, and the President's Award and the Editor's Award from the Wisconsin Medical Credit Association.

With three books on health care financial management to his credit, as well as articles in such journals as the *American Hospital Association Journal*, *Healthcare Financial Management*, *Credit World*, Healthcare Financial Management Association's *Journal of Patient Account Management*, among others, he is an established writer on health care financial management subjects.

INTRODUCTION

In the past few years, medical group practices have seen more change in reimbursement structures than in the previous twenty years. Cost containment at all levels is forcing health insurance carriers to design unique payment packages for the fee-for-service group. We are seeing and will continue to see more deductibles, coinsurance, lifetime maximums, and other reimbursement plans that will change the pattern of payments.

The rapid growth in health maintenance organizations (HMOs), preferred provider organizations (PPOs), and other capitation or discount arrangements will continue to create an interesting mix that will affect the cash flow factor in medical groups. While the capitation reimbursement should be equal to or greater than fee-for-service, it may take two or three years to reach that point. During this interim period, efficient management of accounts receivable will become even more essential.

In addition to the effect of changing reimbursement structures, there is the major impact of a substantial increase in revenue for group practices. An increase in revenue will increase receivables as well as expenses for handling additional patient load within the group. With an increase in expenses, operating profit margins may actually decrease in the early stages, as expenses increase faster than revenues.

For these reasons, efficient management of accounts receivable is more important now than ever before. Effective accounts receivable management will improve the cash flow for a group practice, thereby creating additional investment income and operating revenue.

The twelve key strategies in this book are designed to help medical group practices chart a route to success by maximizing cash flow through proper management of their major asset — accounts receivable.

KEY STRATEGY 1:
DEVELOP CONTROL PRIOR TO SERVICE

One of the key elements to reducing monthly outstanding bookings and improving cash flow in a medical group practice is what is done before service is rendered. An effective previsit registration system is the cornerstone to a successful collection program.

Obtaining Accurate Information

The goal of improving monthly outstanding bookings is greatly enhanced by the acquisition and subsequent use of accurate insurance and financial data on the patient. The gathering of such data is no easy task.

Many people are involved, even the patient's physician under certain circumstances. While everyone tries to work together to get the job done efficiently, there is a practical limit to the type and amount of data that can be collected during a typical preregistration procedure.

Obtaining accurate information is often a task of monumental proportion. For the most part, there is not enough time to get additional data regarding the patient's financial status, not to mention the time required to verify the accuracy of the data obtained. Prior to the day of the appointment or during preregistration is the time to gather data and investigate and isolate problems. The aim should be to preregister between 80 and 90 percent of scheduled new appointments — even if it is only one day prior to the day of service (Hogan).

Advantages of Preregistration for a Group Practice

A preregistration system offers many advantages to a group practice. It can ease the reimbursement process as well as assist personnel with gathering information. Correct and complete information regarding the patient and responsible party can be obtained in a more relaxed setting, on both new and repeat business.

Proper and necessary insurance information can be obtained to verify and bill the patient's insurance carrier, and to avoid unnecessary delays and uneven work flow. The business office will then have up-to-date knowledge of what is needed in the increasingly complex and changing area of health insurance.

A preregistration system affords group practices the opportunity to obtain complete information and to verify insurance benefits by phone and mail as much in advance of the date of service as possible. Groups are in a better position to make sound, unhurried credit judgments based on timely investigations. They are also better able to make financial arrangements to assist the patient in advance of service.

A preregistration system allows groups to program insurance benefits into the computer prior to the patient's visit; thus, fewer errors in coding are made, the work flow is more evenly distributed, there is less confusion, and computer printouts hold more reliable facts.

When designed in a way that familiarizes new patients before the date of service with group services, facilities, and policies, a preregistration system can be useful in enriching the public relations image of a group practice. Patients may view the system as an additional service provided for them by the group.

Advantages of Preregistration for Patients

The patient gains several advantages from a preregistration system as well. The patient spends less time in the registration process the day service is rendered. Crucial information can be keyed into the data processing system prior to the visit, allowing for more time with the physician.

A patient orientation program or preregistration system allows a group's staff to become acquainted with patients and their needs. Patients are more relaxed for their initial visit with the physician, and the staff is consequently better able to serve them and fulfill their needs.

A preregistration visit allows patients to openly discuss financial arrangements in a private area within the group's facility, avoiding an embarrassing situation on the day of service. Patients can plan for the medical costs involved, and rectify past financial problems through counseling in advance of the visit.

A preregistration system permits the obstetrical patient to better understand the financial process and perhaps alleviate some of her financial problems. The obstetrical patient represents the younger population, who often has many current bills and in some cases presents greater collection problems.

Used properly, preregistration can benefit the patient as well as the group practice by conveying policies regarding initial visits, payments, and various other regulations. It is excellent public relations, as well as an effective and necessary information-gathering procedure that can reduce the write-off of bad debts, thus improving collection.

Tips for Developing a Preregistration System

The following guidelines should be kept in mind when setting up a preregistration system:

1. Make preregistration a top priority for everyone, from administration on down.

2. Make it easy for the patient to use preregistration. This means the registration staff should be fully trained in the process.

3. Develop an "upcoming" patient chart for preregistration information. The patient should be contacted forty-eight hours prior to service.

4.   Verify preregistration insurance information prior to service.

5.   Have an estimate of what the patient will owe at time of service, based on his or her verified insurance benefits.

Scheduling and Business Office Liaison

Since many collection problems and misunderstandings crop up after service as a result of improper or inadequate information gathering, it is desirable to have a close liaison between scheduling and business office personnel. First, since the patient information form is used in the same manner as a credit application, needed and accurate information should be gathered during the preregistration procedure. Second, and just as important, the scheduling personnel should be informed about "credit thinking" together with the rest of the business office. Employees' knowledge of credit and collection can be helpful in avoiding future collection problems. When employees know enough about credit and collection, they will obtain extra information, identify potential problems, and pass them on to the credit manager. Credit and collection ignorance is costly. If an employee fails to record essential information accurately or obtains incorrect information, collection problems may arise.

Some large group practices have their business offices check all their scheduled visits against the bad debt file. They then refer repeat offenders to the credit manager. Many items of information are important to the credit manager, and the receptionists or scheduling clerks should obtain these facts. Other group practices have their clerks explain to patients their approximate balance at the time of the visit, inviting the patient to discuss arrangements with the credit manager. Other groups prefer not to discuss money at this time.

By observing important facts presented during preregistration and by obtaining correct information, staff members are more apt to spot potential reimbursement problems and pin them down. In some groups, this is followed up by having the credit manager discuss financial arrangements or by alerting the credit manager shortly after the patient has received the service.

Gathering and relaying necessary credit information is best accomplished by a sympathetic and considerate office staff who consider group practices as service institutions and realize patients visiting physicians are often nervous and apprehensive. While a complete financial statement cannot be expected, adequate information can be diplomatically obtained without causing the patient or the group undue embarrassment.

Staff Training

Often in the past, scheduling personnel have felt they were not a part of the credit and collection operation and innocently neglected to assume proper attitudes toward obtaining necessary information. Also, staff may lack proper training and education in credit and collection procedures and therefore neglect to spot and deal with potential problems.

For better business management within the medical group, consideration should be given to relocating the scheduling office under the same supervision as the collection department and personnel office. Such an organizational system allows managers to train personnel properly in credit and collection procedures that are consistent with good public relations practices.

Trained preregistration personnel will be less likely to overlook essential items such as the correct and full name of the party who is financially responsible for reimbursing the group. Names and addresses of additional family members may be helpful, as are the responsible party's occupation and the name and address of his or her employer. Information of this type can make collection efforts more effective and less time consuming.

Financial Responsibility

Obtaining the signature of someone other than, or in addition to, the patient is important for indication of financial responsibility for medical charges. This has become a bigger issue recently with the increasing number of divorces, separations, and single-parent homes. The most desirable time to obtain the signature is during the preregistration of the patient.

When a person signs acceptance of financial responsibility, but is not legally obligated (someone other than a spouse or parent), the wording of the agreement is of vital importance. If this person is not otherwise legally responsible for the patient's medical bills, an undated, simple statement such as "I agree to pay for services rendered to this patient" may not be sufficient to hold up in court if legal action is taken against the individual signing the ledger or preregistration form. Before the cosigner can be held liable, it is generally upheld that these words must be stated on the medical form: ". . . for and in consideration of acceptance by the XYZ Clinic for services rendered to the patient . . ." To make any type of contract valid, consideration must be given to the party signing and assuming responsibility for reimbursing the group for charges. The safest measure would be to consider including this information the next time medical forms are revised. Sample payment agreements are included in *Figure 1-1*.

Ineffective Preregistration

An ineffective previsit or preregistration system may result in many problems, including the following:

- Lack of understanding of payment policy

- Inefficient and inaccurate collection of vital information required for future communication (such as incorrect spelling of names, addresses, and insurance companies; incomplete addresses; transposed telephone or insurance identification numbers; or failure of patients to bring necessary forms)

- Inadequate knowledge of preauthorization policies

FIGURE 1-1.
SAMPLE PAYMENT AGREEMENTS

SAMPLE 1.

> I/we, the undersigned, do hereby expressly guarantee payment in full of any and all
>
> charges in consideration for medical services rendered, or to be rendered, to
>
> _________________________ by XYZ Clinic commencing _________________, 19____ .
> (patient's name)   (date)
>
> _________________ 19____   X_____________________________________
> (date)   (signature of responsible person)
>
> _________________ 19____   X_____________________________________
> (date)   (signature of responsible person)
>
> Witness _________________________   Address _____________________________

SAMPLE 2.

> **PAYMENT GUARANTEE**
>
> In consideration of acceptance by the clinic of the above named patient and of the
> services rendered and to be rendered to him or her as such patient, the undersigned
> guarantees payment of the account of such patient and agrees to pay the same if not
> paid by the patient at the time of his or her service.
>
> ________________________________   _____________________, 19____
> (signature of responsible person)   (date)

- Failure to collect patient liability at time of service

- Lack of adequate screening and improper evaluation of risks

- Failure to use credit cards when possible

- Failure to take insurance assignments when possible

- Confusion of third-party coverage

- Delay in billing insurance and other third parties

- Inappropriate filing of workers' compensation forms

- Problems in reconciling outstanding monthly bookings

- Lower gross collection ratio

- Greater outstanding receivables

SUMMARY OF KEY STRATEGY 1

In building an overall cash flow strategy for a medical group, a complete previsit and preregistration system should be developed that:

1. Aids in obtaining the information needed to make credit decisions and to bill third-party payers correctly and without delay, both on new and repeat business.

2. Helps in collecting former bad debts or resolving present problems.

3. Signals potentially serious financial losses.

4. Insures that proper signatures are obtained and defines financial responsibility.

5. Is monitored for effectiveness by the person responsible for the accounts receivable and reimbursement process.

KEY STRATEGY 2:
SAFEGUARD CONTROL AT TIME OF SERVICE

Closely connected to effective preregistration procedures and solid medical credit management is a well-organized time-of-service collection process. Sound collection policies begin the day of service.

Reduce the Surprise

Monitoring account balances at the point of service will help reduce the surprise of large balances for both the patient and the practice. Tight controls on payments or keeping tabs on arrangements for the patient's portion of the bill after service has been rendered will go a long way toward keeping the patient's portion of receivables within reasonable limits.

Payment arrangements with the responsible party can sometimes be secured in advance of service in such a way that only the amount owed and the number of payments needed is to be filled in when the patient leaves the clinic. Generally, however, office personnel are confronted with a situation less than ideal. The responsible party may not be available; therefore, needed information cannot be secured.

The After-Service Interview

Group practice personnel agree that certain aspects of the credit interview are more positive than others. The least pleasant tasks that must be accomplished during the interview, of course, deal with the payment due or arrangements for future payment. The interview should develop as positively as possible since this is a critical time for establishing or adding to the rapport between the patient and the medical group.

The need for the cashier or patient account manager to control the interview is obvious. First, patients or responsible parties should be shown the account balance. They need to know the total charges for services. The total should not be kept a deep, dark secret because, really, who has a better right to know than the patient? The patient also should be informed about any untabulated charges, and if an estimate must be made about these, it should be put on the high side.

The next step is to work out the amount of the bill that insurance will cover and to let the patient know how much of the balance will be his or her obligation. It would then be appropriate to ask the patient: "Are you able to pay this amount today?" If cash is forthcoming or a check is written for the full amount, the interview is over for all practical purposes.

It is essential that the interview be completely confidential, with a minimum of interruptions (none, if possible), and that it be conducted in a tactful and diplomatic manner. Open counters are not the best setting. If the cashier becomes impatient, short of answers, or rude, in a few moments, all the good impressions built up during the patient's visit to the medical group may be destroyed. These tactics only succeed in alienating the patient and destroying the image of the group. If the cashier concentrates on the business at hand and deals with the situation in a manner agreeable to the patient, while at the same time fulfilling policy requirements, the group's image will actually be enhanced because of the effort made to work out the problem with the patient.

Sensing Problems Early

The cashier's interview of the patient or the person financially responsible for payment is a critical catch point for increasing collections and reducing later collection problems. It also may help to reduce the number of bad debt write-offs.

If a patient hedges during the interview, there may be a serious problem building. Questions should be asked, and the patient's responses should be closely noted. Perhaps the patient only needs enough time to get the money. On the other hand, there may be a serious financial problem which is aggravated by the need for medical attention.

At this point, the cashier should inform the patient about the group's credit policy regarding payment of accounts. The patient may have already read something about this in the group's brochure. In this way, patients will know how much the group is prepared to do for them. To help patients work out their personal finances, it may be necessary for the medical group to accept the added burden of their medical bills until the patient is better able to pay.

Regardless of whether the group is to carry the account on an installment basis or a note to the bank is to be signed, it is important that the amount of payment (weekly, biweekly, or monthly) is realistic. It is much better to set up a longer payment schedule that the patient can meet than to insist upon higher periodic payments beyond the patient's financial reach. After the necessary paperwork (a note or similar payment agreement) has been signed, the interview is over.

A Last-Chance Situation

The after-service interview could be a last-chance situation. Although the patient or other family member may be returning at a future date, this could be the last convenient opportunity to complete records with information not previously secured. It may be the first and last opportunity to place a bill before the patient and attempt to collect his or her portion.

The policy of securing complete credit information on the day of service is probably even more important when dealing with walk-in patients or unscheduled visitors. Chances are these patients will not return to the medical group for future consultation, and they may not be established patients of this or any other medical group. Many of these patients skip from one medical group to another, never establishing long-term records with any one group.

Records Maintenance

It is a good idea to keep records of accounts collected near the cashiers according to the day and the week of the transaction. Having supervisory personnel screen the previous day's visits will help control loose financial arrangements and identify members of the staff who need additional training in collections. Potential collection problems can also be spotted and forwarded to the manager or collector for immediate follow-up. Data processing reports should be designed to print out the data in a priority sequence for immediate review. Tight control and knowledge of charges and payments are critical to good cash flow.

<table>
<tr><td>SUMMARY OF
KEY STRATEGY 2</td><td colspan="2">Initial control can be safeguarded by designing the following:</td></tr>
<tr><td></td><td>1.</td><td>Monitoring techniques to tabulate prior account balances before the patient is seen again.</td></tr>
<tr><td></td><td>2.</td><td>A follow-up process to complete the payment arrangements agreed upon during the preregistration visit.</td></tr>
<tr><td></td><td>3.</td><td>An interview program for cashiers or collectors to follow during after-service meetings with patients.</td></tr>
<tr><td></td><td>4.</td><td>Flexible reimbursement systems that meet the needs of the patient and fulfill the group's collection policies.</td></tr>
<tr><td></td><td>5.</td><td>A reliable record-keeping system to ensure sound collection facts.</td></tr>
</table>

KEY STRATEGY 3: NEUTRALIZE SMALL BALANCE ACCOUNTS

A continuing problem for medical group managers is collecting the high number of small balance accounts. This deserves special attention because it involves a different kind of accounts receivable problem and should be treated separately in the overall collection strategy. Specific policies, procedures, and techniques should be developed, as well as an overall strategy for controlling and managing the smaller dollar volume in relation to the total account volume. The strategy must allow the staff to spend more time in the profitable areas in order to improve cash flow.

Examination of Present Systems

Only after present collection policies, procedures, and the overall follow-up system have been examined can the necessary adjustments in all three areas be made. Developing a system that can move small balance accounts through a billing cycle to full payment or to a collection agency, with a minimum amount of personal intervention or poor public relations, will go a long way toward establishing a successful cash flow program.

The large number of small balance accounts is one of the biggest headaches for most accounts receivable managers. The personnel time that small balance accounts drain from a group practice can literally destroy all well-meaning goals and plans. These accounts can not only take up all of an employee's time, but also create many public relations problems and offer too little return for time spent. The cost of billing a $20 account is almost identical to the cost of billing a $2,000 account. The savings realized in personnel time with an effective small balance collection system is significant when the system frees collection staff to concentrate on large balance accounts. The result is larger weekly collection totals.

When examining the billing and collection cycle, adjustments can be made to allow for differentiating larger balance accounts from smaller ones. In other words, a system should be developed that will lead to faster conclusions with less effort, especially on balances defined as "small." This is the goal: Neutralize small balance accounts to prevent them from consuming staff time, and use staff time to follow up on large balance accounts.

Different Management Techniques

Nowhere is the expertise of a medical group manager challenged as much as in dealing with the mix of accounts receivable. Regardless of the account characteristics particular to a medical group, the fact remains that different management techniques must be used on small balance accounts if the total accounts receivable balance is to be kept at an acceptable level. Closer examination of specific medical group management techniques reveals those which play an important role in the management of accounts.

Failure to use good management techniques results in a disproportionately high number of small balance accounts becoming uncollectible. These accounts must then be referred to collection agencies for additional collection efforts. Therefore, it is essential to recognize fully the characteristics of the "typical" small balance account and to customize the management techniques used to bring such accounts to a paid-in-full status ("Small Accounts Create Big Collection Problems").

Each medical group may choose to define a small balance account differently. However, the following three traits are generally accepted as typical of small balance accounts:

1.   The account balance is $100 or less.

2.   The account is usually designated as self-pay; that is, the patient or responsible person pays the balance.

3.   Though numerous, together these accounts make up 15 to 20 percent of total receivable dollars outstanding.

Practical Policies

The most important factors of a small balance account collection strategy are practical policies, updated and specific collection procedures, and a unique billing and follow-up system.

First, policies should be developed that are specific to this type of account and separate from large balance account procedures. Patients who cannot or will not pay for services and who have insurance should be asked to assign the benefits of their insurance to the medical group. The insurance company is billed with the understanding that if reimbursement is not received within 45 days, the patient will be billed and payment will be expected at that time. The day the insurance company is billed a copy of the bill should be sent to the patient with a computer-printed message reminding him or her again of the collection policy and of the necessity of sending in the claim forms. The message may read as follows:

"A copy of this bill has been sent to your insurance company."

"Your insurance company may request a claim form from you before it will process your bill for payment. Please complete and return any forms requested from you to your insurance company."

"We will expect payment from either you or your insurance company within 45 days."

Another general statement relating to a specific policy reads:

> "Any medical service not covered by insurance should be paid for at the time of service. No matter how many policies and procedures are developed and followed, an exceptional case will arise. For instance, in an emergency situation, service should be rendered immediately and financial circumstances discussed later. No one should be denied service solely because of lack of money. Because patient account managers are familiar with all phases of credit work and are qualified to set up payment plans to meet a variety of financial circumstances, they are most qualified to work out an agreeable reimbursement plan if an account cannot be paid at the time of service."

Group policies must be practical for small balance accounts and the overall cash flow plan, workable for staff, and adaptable to patient needs. The following policy is recommended: If a patient is found to be a self-pay at the time of registration, payment in full should be requested or a promissory note should be signed and enforced. An itemized statement should be presented at this time. If complete insurance billing information is received at the time of registration, the medical group will bill the account; however, if no payment is received 45 to 60 days after billing, the code is changed to self-pay and the established procedure is followed with no exceptions. If incomplete insurance billing information is received at the time of registration, the account should be coded self-pay and the established procedures should be followed. If this situation occurs and the patient does have adequate coverage, the patient should be held responsible for billing the insurance company. In this case, the patient should be provided with an instruction sheet indicating how insurance forms are to be completed. Should the patient insist that the medical group do the billing, then a fee of $3 to $5 should be requested and paid prior to the completion of the forms.

If cashiers have workable policies to follow, collections will increase, the number of self-pay accounts will go down, and the number of accounts written off to collection agencies will decrease.

Updated and Specific Procedures

Procedures must be updated to fit with policies. Preregistration personnel, as well as the cashier and collectors, need updated and specific procedures.

An account opened properly is half-collected. This familiar credit rule means that when an account is opened according to predetermined steps, it is more likely to be collected in full and without misunderstandings or drawn-out collection procedures. Personnel should not be afraid to ask the necessary questions, but should ask them in a friendly manner. It is not essential to follow the precise order of questions on the registration form; flexibility is often helpful.

In order to collect payment while protecting the patient's dignity, it is good to follow the golden rule: one should behave toward others as one would have others behave toward oneself. At no time should the credit counseling session take on the tone of a business interview. The relationship between patient and professional is too delicate and personal to be put on the same level as a purely business transaction. The needs of the patient must always come first, and a professional approach to human problems should always be maintained.

Rudolph M. Severa, secretary/treasurer of Associated Credit Men of New York and manager of one of the largest credit bureaus in the world, has published a list of ten types of individuals who may be poor risks. The list includes persons, for example, who have no permanent address. Used as a general guide, the points raised by Severa give some idea of the complexity of granting credit. However, it is heartening to note that the vast majority of people are essentially honest and well disposed to paying their bills. Only a minority of people lack the basic characteristics of wholesome and trustworthy citizens.

In gathering information, if the patient is insured, the benefits covered by the patient's insurance company should be reviewed. It is important to note which diagnoses are covered. If the patient has no insurance or is not covered, more information is necessary: What does the patient do for a living? How long has he or she worked at the same job? Where does the patient live? Who is financially responsible? The patient should sign in and include a current address on the registration form. Patient identification should be obtained, and payment in full should be requested on the day of service.

Tips for Collecting at Time of Service

The following guidelines should be kept in mind when collecting at time of service:

1.   Always begin by asking for the balance in full. *"The charge is 'X' dollars. Will that be cash, check, or charge?"* A charge card should be used only if necessary; cash is preferred since it saves time and money.

2.   Sell the importance of paying at time of service.

3.   If the patient cannot pay on the date of service, obtain the date on which the account will be paid in full. Try not to go beyond 30 days.

4.   Develop a sense of urgency with the patient concerning the need for payment in full.

5.   Politely explain that the medical group does not carry accounts without specific prior arrangements.

6.   Ask for identification, including complete name, address, zip code, phone number, and employer's full name.

7.   Ask the self-employed patient what kind of work he or she does.

8.   Get the signature of the financially responsible party.

9.   Obtain and complete, with proper signatures, all credit information.

10.   Always note the date the bill will be paid in full if it cannot be paid on the date of service.

A Unique Billing and Follow-up System

Practical policies and specific procedures for collection at the time of service are critical links to controlling small balance accounts. However, most small balance accounts probably will not be collected at the time of service and will fall into the billing system. This brings us to the third factor in the collection strategy: a unique billing and follow-up system.

The billing and follow-up system for small balance accounts should be specifically geared toward collecting this type of account. A tighter billing cycle will consistently put a statement before the debtor at frequent but reasonable intervals. Consideration also should be given to varying the wording on subsequent notices to make them different from initial statements. The idea is to send out a series of notices (three or four) within a short period of time. After this period of time, the bill can be sent to an agency or telephone contact may be made if staff is available. Various billing cycles are illustrated in *Figure 3-1*.

FIGURE 3-1.
BILLING CYCLES

Plan	Days Between Notices	Billing Cycle Item
Plan 1:	30 days	Initial statement
	10 days	Second statement
	10 days	Third statement
	10 days	Review
	10 days	Final notice
		After 70 days send to agency
Plan 2:	30 days	Initial statement
	15 days	Second statement
	15 days	Third statement
	10 days	Review
	10 days	Final notice
		After 80 days send to agency
Plan 3:	30 days	Initial statement
	30 days	Second statement
	15 days	Third statement
	10 days	Review
	10 days	Final notice
		After 95 days send to agency
Plan 4:	30 days	Initial statement
	15 days	Second statement
	15 days	Review
	10 days	Final notice
		After 70 days send to agency

No attention, no collection! Specific advice on designing notices to draw attention (including information on size, motion, isolation, color, and legibility) is provided in Key Strategy 7. At the least, notices should command and hold sufficient attention for the entire message to be read. A billing cycle set up over a 70- to 95-day period with well-designed notices that prompt results, together with an effective system to cover third-party insurance and self-pay accounts, encapsulates the total strategy.

Cycles that provide the options of a collection agency, write-off, or phone work within 70 to 95 days will improve the collection ratio and improve cash flow. More importantly, effective collection at the time of service and a quick billing cycle with notices that pack a punch will allow staff to spend more time on large balance accounts. One of the secrets for decreasing outstanding monthly balances is to concentrate attention on accounts that create the majority of the total outstanding receivables. An example of a total collection system is provided in *Figure 3-2*.

FIGURE 3-2.
A TOTAL COLLECTION SYSTEM

- Charges not covered by insurance are payable upon completion of service.

- Billing
  - Prepare and mail initial bill to insurance or patient within seven days of service.
  - Utilize data mailers and/or notices:
    - Uninsured Patients
      - Send three or four reminder statements within 95 days.
      - Prelist with agency at 100 to 120 days from last date of service.
      - Include this message in final notice: "Going to collection agency within seven days."
      - Agency write-off at 120 days.
    - Insured patients
      - Starting at 45 days, send three reminder statements to the patient within the 75 days following. Specific samples of messages to be used on statements are provided in Key Strategy 7.
      - Prelist on computer as bad debt at 90 days after sending the initial statement with final notice and message.
      - Start listing as bed debt automatically at 120 days after initial reminder.

- Collection
  - Phone follow-up starts on accounts over $100 with no insurance at 45 days.
  - Balances under $100 go through system without phone work.

- Write-off
  - Develop billing statements and messages with punch and a time sequence that is tight.
  - Keep bad debt prelist at 90 days from initial statement and write-off at 120 days. Accounts without payment should not be kept in open receivables beyond that point.
  - Concentrate more collection effort at time of service by firming up credit arrangements. Eliminate problems before they start.
  - Send statements first, then have phone collectors work the account. Concentrate all collection phone work on accounts that appear on the prelist.

Managing small balance accounts requires the use of customized collection techniques. In most cases, a manager does not have enough time to become familiar with the patient, to verify the correctness of all patient information received, to make formal payment arrangements, and to become assured of the timely collection of the account. However, when practical policies and specific procedures are adopted for use with small balance accounts and followed by the collection staff, the patient accounts manager will be in a better position to control this portion of the medical group's cash flow. The amount of time spent on small balance accounts will be minimized, and more time can be devoted to larger balance accounts.

**SUMMARY OF
KEY STRATEGY 3**

In building the overall collection system for a medical group, a small balance collection strategy should be developed that:

1. Is tied to a specific policy.

2. Has specific procedures.

3. Emphasizes collection at time of service for small balance accounts.

4. Has a special billing cycle and statement sequence for fast turnaround to paid status, agency, or write-off.

5. Incorporates maximum recovery of small balance accounts while pushing them through the system with minimal staff time and effort, thus allowing more follow-up time for large balance accounts.

KEY STRATEGY 4:
IMPROVE STAFF ABILITY TO COLLECT

Collection in medical groups is more important today than it has ever been. A large number of factors in the environment have placed health care providers in a cash flow situation that simply demands a faster turnaround of payment. By the same token, it has become equally important to maintain favorable public relations during the collection process so that patients are not lost to the competition.

In the middle of this situation sit the employees who function as collectors. While sitting on a "hot seat," they make a sizable contribution to the financial success and the public relations image of a medical group. However, too often employees in collector positions are underqualified and underpaid, and there are not enough of them to get the job done.

Underqualified Collectors

Few medical group employees have previous collection experience at a bank, finance company, or similar consumer credit company. Too often, they simply do not know how to collect.

Poorly qualified health care collectors tend to set up financial arrangements that prolong payment, rather than take the steps necessary to accelerate the turnaround of receivables. Collectors with an inadequate collection background can become easy prey for clever debtors and slow-paying insurance companies.

One way to improve cash flow is to hire good collectors and then train, train, train. It is the manager's job to hire high-quality people and conduct the training for this key position. When screening applicants for collector positions, it is important to look for certain traits. Top candidates are those with natural ability, a pleasant personality, strong common sense, and who are logical and presentable to the public. When an applicant is found who has these qualities as well as some type of credit and collection background in either finance, retail, or wholesale, it is time to make a selection.

Underpaid Collectors

Unfortunately, collectors in medical groups are often underpaid compared to their peers in banks, finance companies, retail stores, and collection agencies. While money is not always a motivator, low salaries do not attract the best, and many will go elsewhere to achieve higher status.

In addition to the lower salaries, collector bonuses are almost unheard of in medical groups although they are quite common in other organizations dealing in consumer collection. Collection bonus programs can be more than just a means to increase overall collection volume. Managers can adapt incentive plans to achieve specific revenue and profit objectives. At the same time, incentives can inject new energy into the collection effort by offering collectors prestige as well as tangible rewards. With a well-designed program, a medical group practice can attract and retain top producers as well as motivate average performers to excel.

After specific goals are established, the next step is to decide what results will be rewarded so that efforts can be channeled in the appropriate direction. Some managers structure their collection incentive programs to reward in these areas:

- Highest dollar volume collected

- Greatest percentage increase in dollars collected (to motivate improved performance)

- Highest volume collected each day (to maintain ongoing enthusiasm)

- Greatest percentage of reduction in accounts receivable

- Longest period during which collection quotas are met (to sustain effort)

It is often advantageous to set collection goals in terms of percentages, rather than in units or dollars. For example, collectors in their first year may be discouraged by dollar amounts. In fact, there is little that can be done to equalize the program for newcomers when unit volume is the only goal. Structuring incentives based on percentages can motivate new collectors.

Another consideration is that not every veteran collector will react in the same way to a given incentive. Top performers typically excel without a bonus program, while poor performers may not improve significantly even with additional incentives. In setting goals, therefore, the key is to motivate average performers. This is the group whose collections are most likely to increase with the introduction of an incentive. Further, the ability to motivate average performers, as well as new people, depends largely on the rewards selected.

A properly implemented incentive program based on collections will increase employee motivation. A combination of team and individual incentives will provide the best results. In this way, the team concept is promoted, while individual excellence is recognized.

Not Enough Collectors

The cure for high receivables and slow cash flow is — collectors. This is one case where more is better. Most medical groups do not put enough people in the collection process. With the increase in patient liability due to changes in insurance payment today, practices are becoming buried in self-pay accounts. Having enough well-paid, efficient collectors has always been important, but now it is vital.

Having more top-notch collection personnel and offering them incentives will lead to lower days outstanding. National surveys consistently show those participating providers with the lowest days outstanding had twice the number of collectors as providers with the highest days outstanding. Developing a collection staff with a good ratio of full-time equivalent (FTE) employees to open accounts and with a decent pay scale has become of paramount importance to medical group managers

What is a good standard to use for determining how many collectors should be hired? Several factors influence the ideal standard, including the following:

- **Percentage of self-pay.** The larger the number of self-pay accounts, the larger the number of collectors needed. Other third-party payer mixes will also dictate need.

- **Present days outstanding.** If days outstanding are presently over 70, more collectors will be needed to pull down this figure.

- **Effective financial control at time of service.** If a high percentage of patients pay at the time of service, fewer collectors will be needed.

Auditing Collector Effectiveness

Too often we complain that we do not have enough collectors to get the job done. This may well be the case. However, how effective are the ones we have? Are they working at maximum productivity? How do we really know? An audit of the effectiveness of each collector should be conducted by the supervisor on a regular basis, and by the medical group manager once every couple of months.

First, thorough collection notations by collectors should be mandatory. A good audit cannot be conducted unless all collection activity is dated and noted. In reviewing accounts on which the collector has been working, the following observations should be made:

1. When is the collection follow-up started? Is procedure being followed? For instance, is follow-up on a large balance commercial account begun 30 days from billing, or some time much later? When is follow-up begun on the self-pay financial classes for which the collector is responsible?

2. Is full payment or partial payment received for self-pay accounts? Are small monthly payments accepted too easily?

3. Are insurance personnel giving the collector the runaround? Does the collector appear to be getting delays and put-offs when he or she follows up on the insurance classifications? Constant call-backs and lack of reason for delays should be noted. Is the collector trying to settle quickly or accepting the easy way out too often?

4. Are there too many "no answers"? Contact notations of "no answer" on self-pay accounts should be reviewed. This indicates the need to call at night or some other time when the patient is at home.

5.   Are there too many notations? Is there too much follow-up activity by the collector on a consistent basis? If most accounts have many contacts, it is a sign of losing the battle. The collector is getting pushed around and delayed, or else lacks the skills or initiative to get the account paid.

6.   Is there prompt follow-up? For those accounts requiring collection follow-up on a previous promise, collection calls should be made on the date of the promise, not days or weeks later.

Listening to collection calls offers another means of evaluating collector effectiveness. A phone arrangement that allows directly listening to the conversations of collectors, or if that is not possible, at least sitting nearby and listening to some calls, may provide valuable information. The length of time on the telephone, how put-offs and delays are handled, and persistence should be noted, as well as public relation skills while collecting.

A productivity/time study is also helpful. In this type of study, collectors are required to keep track of their time for a two-week period, identifying what they did by 15-minute increments for the entire time they are on the job. The number of outgoing and incoming collection calls (contacts only) made during each 15-minute period is recorded. The productivity/time sheets are collected at the end of each day, and findings are summarized at the end of the two-week period: What is the average number of calls in and out per day? How are collectors spending their time? Are they performing too many non-collecting functions which cut into their effectiveness as collectors? A sample collector review form is provided in *Figure 4-1*.

Regular audits provide the information necessary to coach collectors to better performance. They clearly indicate the areas that need improvement. After an audit, the emphasis should be on coaching staff into "collectors" of payment instead of "recorders" of the reasons accounts are not getting paid. After all, the bottom line is money, not notations.

To ensure collectors are performing up to the set standards, the following performance indicators should be tracked and analyzed:

- Dollars collected by financial class according to collector responsibility
- Aged trial balance by financial class
- Percentage of receivables over 90 days old
- Bad debt percentage by collector responsibility

Managers should review these key performance reports at least monthly and maybe even on a weekly basis. The point is to analyze data frequently enough to take action when the information does not seem right or when troublesome trends are beginning to take shape.

Tracking critical areas, analyzing data regularly, and taking necessary action is the management combination for a faster turnaround of receivables.

FIGURE 4-1.
COLLECTOR REVIEW FORM

Collection Task	8 - 9	9 - 10	10 - 11	11 - 12	12 - 1	1 - 2	2 - 3	3 - 4	4 - 5

NOTE: Please record <u>all</u> incoming and outgoing phone calls made or received in the space provided below:

	8 - 9	9 - 10	10 - 11	11 - 12	12 - 1	1 - 2	2 - 3	3 - 4	4 - 5
Incoming Calls									
Outgoing Calls									

Developing Good Collectors

Developing good collectors is a critical part of the medical group manager's job. So much is at stake as a result of the performance of collectors. Successful managers constantly work with their collectors to develop a winning attitude that says, "I am a professional, my position is important, and I will be successful." Collectors should be encouraged to:

1.   Develop their own qualities.
2.   Improve their collection techniques.
3.   Continually indulge in self-development.

4.   Practice good human relations skills.
5.   Develop sound work habits.

The first and most important steps in development, according to successful managers, are a positive job attitude, sound work habits, and a goal for the future.

Training collectors in collection techniques consistent with favorable patient relations is the key to successful receivables management in a medical group practice. If collectors can improve their skills by just 10 percent, or improve collection totals by 10 percent, this makes a significant contribution to the total recovery effort. Individual collections in the follow-up process are critical to the total collection strategy. Therefore, time is well spent training collectors in techniques to help them in one-on-one collection situations, as well as in the "art" of collecting.

Any individual who intends to collect medical bills should learn at the outset that collection, much like the practice of medicine, is an art and not an exact science. As an art, it cannot be learned quickly nor can it be practiced in a mechanical or indifferent way. A health care collector must learn the symptoms of the case before a course of treatment can be planned and carried out.

Good collectors must learn to talk to people and be inquisitive enough to find out their motives for acting one way or another under particular conditions. They must be able to communicate their thinking and reasoning in order to motivate the debtor to make payment.

Building a Game Plan

Building an overall game plan for collection calls can be profitable. In working to develop staff collection calls into more productive efforts, it is wise to draw up both "offensive" and "defensive" plans of collection.

The following offensive guidelines should be kept in mind by collectors:

- **Do not prolong a collection call with conversational chatter.** Terminate it as soon as possible while maintaining good public relations techniques.

- **Do not argue.** Some angry patients come through with payment after venting all their anger on you. Others, when they fail to arouse you, have no defenses left.

- **Use intelligence, not emotion.** The collector's approach must be dispassionate and logical rather than social or emotional. The collector is an agent of society trying to insure that individuals honor their contracts. Even though the collector may be sympathetic to an individual debtor, he or she must remember the responsibility of the medical group to the other patients who pay their bills on time.

- **Sound confident and mature.** Communicate authority, and command respect.

- **Use a businesslike manner.** Treat matters seriously, and state facts with conviction and assurance. Be friendly, but not familiar. Firmness is more convincing when coupled with a formal tone.

- **Be courteous.** Maintain dignity and decorum. Be firm without ever being vulgar.

- **Be flexible in your approach if the situation warrants it.** If it is necessary to become more firm, you can "put a chill in the air" without becoming nasty or unpleasant. On the other hand, you may wish to sympathize and use warmth without being too personal.

- **Be natural.** Use simple, uncomplicated sentences. Make your delivery unhurried and deliberate.

It is to the collector's advantage to make the first move. At the outset of the call, the collector should identify himself or herself and the organization, state what the call is about, mention the balance due, and then wait. It is not necessary to go into arguments or persuasion. It is not necessary to mention previous efforts to collect. The conversational vacuum should not be filled up by the collector; rather, he or she should just wait for a response. The debtor's reaction will tell a lot about how to approach the situation. Tips for responding to common debtor defenses are outlined below:

- **Aggression and attack.** An unexpected call and its timing may create an emergency in the mind of the debtor, and he or she may attack by complaining (often unjustly) about services. Do not defend! The best tactic is to express pleasure at knowing the cause of the delay and a willingness to make adjustments in order to correct the problem.

  It is important to get a commitment from the patient to send all the facts by a certain date. If the complaint is legitimate, it should be corrected. If it is a stall, the collector should make it difficult for this defense to continue. It is hard for the debtor to fight someone who meets belligerence with cooperation and pleasantness.

- **Pleas for sympathy.** Be it true or false, the story must not be disputed. Sympathy should be expressed, as well as persistence for payment. If the patient is in real trouble and an extension is granted, the matter must not be treated lightly. Stress the seriousness. The terms of repayment should be specific, and these should be impressed upon the debtor.

- **Denial and evasion.** Some debtors deny knowledge of a debt. Do not try to prove them wrong; this would be unprofessional. Rather, the debtor must be given every opportunity to claim the debt. State the facts: dates, reason for the visit, physician's name, and so on. Then, request immediate payment. If this defense is used once, more of the same may be expected. The patient may promise payment, but fail to follow through. This type of excuse is a cover for the real reason for nonpayment.

- **Defiance**. The debtor may say, "So what?" Maintain your composure and keep command of the situation. Remain cool and polite. Make a direct request for payment, but do not argue. When a collector refuses to argue, the debtor may continue to press an aggressive attack and reveal the true motives for his or her behavior. If the debtor simply refuses to pay at all, calmly and politely state that if payment is not made by a certain date in the near future, claim will be placed for collection.

The collection call may be a threat to a debtor's self-esteem or a threat to security. Some will run by lying or postponing, others will slug it out by fighting, arguing, or expressing sarcasm.

Questioning Techniques

The number one rule in successful collections is: People prefer talking to listening. No doubt about it — the person who talks intelligently about a number of different subjects does not make the same impression as the person who asks you a number of intelligent questions and listens to what you have to say.

The ability to ask questions is essential to successful collections. Patients give a variety of excuses for not paying, and often the excuses they give are a cover-up of the real reason they are not paying. Questions may be helpful in sorting through excuses and real objections.

Questions also allow the collector to keep control of a collection call. When asking questions, a leader role is established, and the conversation may be guided where the collector wants it to go.

It is helpful to use questions that begin with who, what, when, where, and why. These types of questions require an expansive response from the patient. By prompting the patient to say more than "yes" or "no", valuable information for understanding the situation may be elicited. However, in the case of a patient who rambles quite a bit, yes/no questions may keep the patient on track.

Questions can be used to motivate payment. Changing current motivational phrases into questions will usually yield better results. For instance, a popular motivational phrase is: "If you don't pay, your account will go to a collection agency." The word "if" implies a threat: "If you don't do this, something bad will happen." Even the implication of a threat will get a poor response from patients. Instead, the same motivator may be phrased as a question: "You don't want your account to go to a collection agency, do you?" This requires the patient to respond and is less threatening, even though it implies the same thing.

All statements can be phrased as questions, right? Any phrases or statements currently used to motivate patients can easily be turned into a question for a better response, can't they? Practice making all statements into questions for one day in order to get in the habit of using questions, okay? This will improve collection techniques tremendously, won't it?

Questions find out what will motivate payment. Questions will uncover the facts and reveal the reason the patient or insurance company is not paying. Questions should be asked until the underlying objection to payment has been discovered.

A picture can be painted in the mind of the patient by using questions. The following examples illustrate how to use questions to paint a picture and motivate payment:

"Won't it be great to get this off your mind?"

"Won't it be great to keep your line of credit clean?"

"Isn't a good credit rating worth $250?"

"This is really what you want, isn't it?"

"Would you rather talk with our attorney?"

Questions in the choice technique are also valuable. Statements tell patients what to do, and nobody likes to be told what to do. Instead, patients can be asked what they would like to do by using the choice technique:

"Would you like to pay today, or should I give you until the end of the month?"

"Do you want to pay by cash, check, or credit card?"

"Can you drop the payment in the mail today, or would you like to stop by the office this afternoon?"

Giving patients the choice of how they will pay in full will yield great results. However, it is important to remember that all of the choices must be in favor of the medical group.

"No" is a forbidden word. This is a very easy word to use, so collectors must be careful that questions do not give patients a chance to say "no" to paying. For example, when a patient is asked, "Will you be sending payment today?" it is setting up a response of "no." It is much more productive to ask, "When will you be sending payment?" or to use the choice technique described above.

Using questions effectively is one of the most effective collection tools available. Questions break the indifference barrier. A top-flight collector can carry through the whole collection call from beginning to end, making no statements and using only questions. In the words of Rudyard Kipling:

> I keep six honest serving men
> (They taught me all I knew);
> Their names are What and Why and When
> And How and Where and Who.

FIGURE 4-2.
MOTIVATOR TOPICS FOR COLLECTING

Topic	Reasoning
Good credit rating	Make debtors realize that good credit is their most valuable asset.
Honesty and reputation	Dwell on their reliability and reputation for fair play.
Freedom from worry	Show debtors how to relieve their minds of worry and protect their credit ratings.
Appreciation	Tell them that arrangements have been made as a favor to them; they can show their appreciation by paying.
Added costs	Ask debtors to pay today to avoid additional costs, and explain that additional charges will be added if legal action is taken. Do not threaten unless you are ready to carry out your promise.*
Avoid trouble	Explain that if payment is not received, there is no alternative but to give the account to a professional collection agency and they can well imagine the trouble this could cause them. Be specific in creating a fear motive, or use fear of the unknown which can also be a tremendous motivator.*

** Be cautious about making threats or creating fear. Consult your attorney.*

The Lombardi Rules

Vince Lombardi, famous coach of the Green Bay Packers, was featured in a 1968 management and sales film entitled *Second Effort*. The film illustrates how the application of some fundamental principles that Lombardi sees as essential for championship football could also apply to the sales field. The lessons gleaned from Lombardi's winning philosophy can apply directly to the art of improving collection results.

Lombardi stressed five main motivators that will produce a winning combination:

1. Develop mental toughness.
2. Control the ball.
3. Stay in shape.
4. Use time wisely.
5. Make that second effort.

Develop mental toughness.   Mental toughness is a keystone of the Lombardi philosophy. He stated, "You carry on no matter what the obstacles. You simply refuse to give up. When the going gets tough, you get tougher. You refuse to let failures — or anything, or anyone — get you down."   This principle views 75 percent of success as a mental process.   In other words, the individual best mentally prepared wins.

Mental preparation includes recognizing and knowing opponents and preparing for them. In collection, the following individuals generally are viewed as opponents:

- **Others**. These may include debtors, an insurance company, or others.

- **Ourselves**. We are sometimes filled with pessimism, negativism, laziness, self-doubt, and complacency.

- **Other medical groups**. They are the competition in outstanding bookings and bad debt write-offs.

- **Time**. We are always trying to beat the clock.

"If success is 75 percent mental," Lombardi said, "we have to be more mentally prepared than our opponents during competition." The first step in this preparation is to know and understand the debtor better. This includes knowing how to collect more effectively, and how to concentrate and refresh one's self and staff on the basics of collection. Commercial insurance companies, their personnel, and their methods of payment should be studied in depth. An attempt must be made to eliminate all hurdles and obstacles regarding payment. Adequate time should be taken to study and thoroughly understand Blue Cross/Blue Shield, Medicare, and Medicaid, their processing methods, and payment procedures. What ties up these accounts? They are obvious opponents, and it is well worth the time to get to know them as thoroughly as possible. Success in collection is dependent upon knowledge of these "others."

We ourselves become opponents to success by making errors, by being careless, by our own lack of order and organization, and by not revitalizing poor systems and inadequate procedures. We also have mental hurdles to overcome — pessimism and negativism, among others. Lombardi said, "We lick these opponents by developing mental toughness within ourselves through sacrifice, self-denial, refusing to give in to ourselves, knowing our job, and dedication and determination to perform our best effort." In the end, we have to provide the stimulus ourselves. Self-discipline is the personal motivation and the necessary effort in which the will determines the objective, method, and desired goals. Lombardi defined mental toughness as the perfectly disciplined will. "You discipline your will," he said, "by refusing to give in to yourself."

The collector and the medical group manager are judged by performance. With mental toughness, attention is concentrated on every small detail of the job, with a determination to have one's best traits working in every way at all times.

Mental toughness is a state of mind, one that refuses to admit defeat. It could almost be called character in action. Roadblocks thrown in the way of a collector with mental toughness are a stimulant rather than a depressant. They are challenging. One of the greatest contributions that mental toughness makes to a manager is confidence; confidence so firm and strong that is simply cannot be overcome. Good physical condition contributes to good mental condition, of course, but the major factor to securing mental toughness is self-confidence.

Control the ball. The great coach said that the only reason his teams ever lost a game is that time ran out on them. The key to success is to control the ball for as many plays as possible. Collectors have a great many points they must make to promptly settle accounts. If they skip any of them, it may be the one payment that will obtain the debtor's payment in full. As a collector, the only way to be sure of making every pertinent collection point is to keep control of the conversation. In football, the team that controls the ball controls the game. In collecting, the collector who controls the conversation brings home the balance.

Skilled collectors direct everything that happens during a collection call. If collectors feel that they are about to lose the ball, they make a quick analysis and alter the collection approach to fit the situation. There are numerous "option plays" to maintain control of the ball. We can apply that principle by realizing that one way to control the ball is to know the job more completely. Knowing every detail of our job better than anyone else competing for the debtor's dollars or the insurance payment puts us in control of the situation.

Collectors must have extensive knowledge of their medical group's terms and charges, and credit and collection procedures and policies so that questions can be answered promptly and with authority. In addition, the more we know about the debtor and the insurance companies, the more we will be able to face and control any situation. Another way to control the ball is by taking the initiative, taking command, and not allowing efforts to be blocked.

Stay in shape. "Fatigue makes cowards of us all." Good physical condition breeds self-confidence, and confidence breeds success. The main focus is to stay in shape. The strain and pressures of the job demand that collection personnel be in top shape. This motivator may well be the cornerstone to all the rest.

Anyone who thinks about it for even a few seconds realizes that a professional who is in good physical condition can perform more efficiently. When someone is tired physically, he or she is tired mentally, too. Drive and aggressiveness are lacking. Lombardi believed that a person who is physically fit is able to perform better at any job. To the dedicated professional, physical fitness means more than a suggestion to follow a regular regimen of sit-ups. It means proper diet, and it means getting as much sleep as necessary to restore the body to peak efficiency after a hard day's work.

Good use of time. Ron Kramer, who became an all-time football great under Lombardi's training, once said, "There's regular time and Lombardi time. With Lombardi time, if you're ten minutes early for practice, you're still late." Lombardi time goes far beyond being punctual about appointments. His squads worked longer and harder than most, and every minute of every hour in every working day was perfectly planned to get maximum results. Lombardi time utilizes every second.

Collectors are limited in the volume they can produce by the number of working hours in a day. Actually, in many cases, a collector is forced to compress collection efforts into a very few hours. Since collectors are judged by collection results and there are only certain hours when collections can be made, every minute must be utilized to maximize effectiveness. Considering two collectors of equal ability, if one budgets for maximum collection time and makes 20 more calls per week than the other, the weekly comparison record will certainly reflect the greater effectiveness.

Time spent for a "call back" when one call should have done the job is not Lombardi time. Time spent on a collection call with inadequate preparation is not Lombardi time.

Make that second effort. This was Lombardi's favorite motivator. The meaning is simple enough: If you get stalled, shift gears, make a second effort, take the initiative. Force the opponent to make a decision. Don't give in. Go that extra step. Make each call the one that will make today's goal in the collection total. Don't get stopped on the one-yard line when you should be scoring.

Lombardi never gave an opponent an inch, yet he also stressed respect for the dignity of the opponent. In his case, it was the other team. In the collector's case, it is the people with whom he or she is talking or dealing. It should be kept clearly in mind that they are the ones who are trying to block the goal of collection. They are the "competition." We must really dig in and continue to study how to deal with people. This should never be considered too fundamental. Although they are the competition, we must learn to respect and understand them. Human dignity can never, never be sacrificed for personal success.

Lombardi said, "I have to sell my players on themselves, on forgetting the small hurts because they're a part of life. I have to sell them on making this team, this season, this game, and each individual play the most important thing in their lives. I ask them to live up to their potential. If you don't do that, whether you're playing football or selling, you're a cheat. You're a cheat to yourself and to your company."

SUMMARY OF KEY STRATEGY 4

Collection totals will only be as good as the people collecting. Improving the skills and the performance of collectors is the key to improving the total collection system. When developing a collection program, the following areas should be considered:

1. The performance of collectors will make a sizable contribution to the financial success and public relations of a medical group.

2. A properly implemented incentive program based on collections will increase employee motivation.

3. By tracking and auditing the performance of collectors on a regular basis, information will be gathered that will prove valuable for coaching collectors to a superior performance.

4. Training collectors on collection techniques consistent with favorable public relations is essential to successful management of a practice.

5. Collectors must be taught how to organize their collection "offenses," and how to recognize the debtor's "defenses."

6. It should always be kept in mind that the job of collectors is to collect, sell, and motivate — not downgrade and humiliate.

7. Incorporating effective questioning techniques into the collection approach will produce positive results.

8. The "Lombardi rules" can be useful in guiding collection staff to success.

KEY STRATEGY 5: CONCENTRATE COLLECTION EFFORTS ON INSURANCE

Insurance collections involve many of the same one-on-one techniques covered in Key Strategy 4. However, there is enough of a difference in third-party recovery to devote a separate strategy to the subject. Since the majority of outstanding receivables is tied up in third-party collections, the overall strategy developed here will play a major role in improving cash flow and reducing the monthly outstanding balance to three months or less.

Before and After

In third-party reimbursement, what is done before the service is rendered is as important as what is done after the bill has been created. Obtaining correct information is as critical as follow-up. Also, knowledge of the major insurance companies' staffs, procedures, and requirements has become essential to third-party reimbursement. An insurance process should be established that is centered around two main strategies: (1) initial data collection, and (2) a state-of-the-art billing and follow-up system.

- **Initial data collection.** The collection of good insurance billing data starts in the preregistration program, at registration, or during the patient's visit. There is no good excuse for not getting proper billing data at one of these points.

- **State-of-the art billing system.** In today's reimbursement environment, quickly producing a clean claim to the third-party payer is critical. Use of electronic claims processing which passes third-party edits is the key to a state-of-the-art billing system. If electronic billing is not used, tight control in the billing section is the next focus of attention. Billing statements should go out as soon and as accurately as possible. The most efficient way to attain this end is to monitor the daily output of each biller and compare it to the goal.

Various information reports can be useful for monitoring the extent of the billing staff's activity. Every attempt should be made to maintain timely control of billing and follow-up. With a schedule and a manager willing to put in the effort necessary to make it work, excellent control can be achieved (Dingess, 1983).

Electronic Claims Processing

Electronic claims processing is the electronic submission of claims to clearinghouses which reformat the claim data and retransmit it to the appropriate insurance company or fiscal intermediary. There are many companies offering some aspect of electronic claims processing, most of them selling software that provides an electronic format for paper claims. There are three major types of electronic claims processing vendors:

1. **Blue Cross/Blue Shield plans.** Generally, the Blue Cross/Blue Shield plans account for the largest electronic claims volume and the longest running operation.

2. **Third-party clearinghouses.** Third-party clearinghouses are vendors who edit and even fix claims so they can get paid by the third parties.

3. **Software vendors.** There are literally hundreds of medical software vendors from which to choose. A current listing entitled *Directory of Software Vendors for Group Practice* can be obtained by contacting the Library Resource Center of the Medical Group Management Association (Herrin, 1992).

Whichever vendor is chosen, electronic claims processing offers these advantages:

- Ability to edit (and then correct) claims prior to submission to the third-party payer

- System-generated productivity reports

- Significant reduction in the number of rebillings

However, it is important to understand that electronic billing does not solve all billing problems. Poor upfront information gathering or slow charge posting will hurt the effectiveness of electronic billing.

Billing Control Reports

Whether or not electronic billing is used, reports designed to monitor a billing staff can provide valuable information and help achieve control. A daily billing control sheet is one example. A form is completed and submitted daily by each biller. On it is recorded the number of bills received by each biller (segregated by financial class) and the number of bills sent for payment. The number entered by the biller as the number of payments received represents the bills given to the biller that morning by the distribution designee. The billers are to submit these forms to the department manager at the end of each day. If a data processing program is developed that captures the same information, it will save employee time and provide more accurate data. The purpose of this report is to monitor the backlog of bills to be completed by the billing staff. If an automated billing system is in place, this control report would not be necessary. A sample daily billing control sheet is provided in *Worksheet 1* in Appendix A.

Another valuable report is a monthly compilation of the daily billing control sheet figures. Combining daily report totals into a monthly summary sheet enables managers to define collection and biller trends on a continuous basis. This report also allows managers to monitor assignment distribution to billers, total billing in each category, and outgoing billings per month. A sample monthly billing control report is provided in *Worksheet 2* in Appendix A.

Still another billing control form can be designed to monitor the unbilled accounts designated as "backlog" on the daily billing control sheet. A sample weekly unbilled insurance report is provided in *Worksheet 3* in Appendix A.

The manager should determine if the number of bills received, as reported by the biller on the daily billing control sheet, is the same as the number reported as distributed to the biller. This will reflect whether the biller is reporting accurate information. Also, the number of bills sent for payment as reported by each biller should be reasonably comparable to the number received. This can vary a bit due to delays in receiving accounts or proper coding of diagnosis and procedures.

Periodically, the cumulative results of this report should be discussed with those employees who are not performing satisfactorily, whether in conjunction with their completion of the daily billing control sheet or in overall evaluation of their productivity. Therefore, in addition to the useful billing information supplied by this production schedule, there is a long-range psychological benefit. A schedule such as this will let productive workers know their work is being recognized. At the same time, nonproductive workers will see that their deficiencies will no longer go unobserved or unaddressed (Dingess, 1983).

A practical strategy is to split the billing by assigning each billing staff member a different portion of the alphabet and letting staff members bill to every type of financial class or category. This gives more coverage during vacations, illnesses, turnovers, and days off, and it provides a more balanced workload for billing staff. It also furnishes comprehensive statistics for comparison and creates competition among staff members.

Effective Follow-Up Policy

The key to third-party claims reimbursement is an effective follow-up policy. In order to be effective, follow-up activities must be consistent and persistent. Being consistent means complying with the policy on a regular basis and keeping exceptions to a minimum. Being persistent means being firm with insurance company personnel and not accepting stalls or delays (Ibid.).

Managers have been given many reasons over the years for claim payment delays. Some of the most commonly reported are:

- Claim never received
- Claim "pending" with no real reason for the delay
- Insurance claim form not completed properly
- Primary insurer must pay first
- Additional medical record information needed
- Coverage questionable
- No employer claimant statement
- No assignment of benefits

- Insurance company computer conversion problems
- Insurance company computer broken down
- Claims sent to corporate office for review

Telephone calls are the best means of following up with insurance carriers today. Most insurance company personnel will not respond to letters immediately; sometimes they will not respond at all. A telephone call demands an immediate response. Proven follow-up techniques by major financial class are provided in *Figure 5-1*.

FIGURE 5-1.
PROVEN FOLLOW-UP TECHNIQUES BY MAJOR FINANCIAL CLASS

Payer	Best Follow-Up Techniques
Blue Cross/Blue Shield	Phone follow-up is best. However, edit reports such as a work-in-progress report are an effective way to monitor unpaid claims.
Commercial	Phone follow-up is always the best approach. Get the patient involved early in the collection process. Save the tracers for the small balance accounts.
HMO/PPO	Phone follow-up is preferred. An aged trial balance (ATB) listing of outstanding claims by each HMO or PPO is another effective method of getting paid (past the contractual obligation of the HMO or PPO).
Medicare	Similar to Blue Cross/Blue Shield. Phone contact works best. However, edit reports such as a work-in-progress report are an effective way to follow up on unpaid claims.
Medicaid	Phone follow-up is best (if contact can be made). "Claims pending" reports generated by the Medicaid system are also a good way to monitor unpaid claims.

Preparation and Contact

The key to successful telephoning is preparation. Files should be reviewed to determine whether previous calls have been made or letters have been sent with no response. If a contact cannot be made, the file should be placed on hold and called back in a few days. Or, if a "return call" message is left with an insurance company representative and there is no response, a call back should be made at another time. It is important not to ignore an account because a call cannot be made that day or at that particular time. Telephone calls previously made, letters that have been sent, additional bills, or additional information that has already been forwarded to the insurance company should be made known to the insurance company representative.

There are several steps that can be taken to follow up on most types of payment delays. They are not new; many successful managers have been practicing these techniques for years. Assuming a claim has been filed accurately and properly, with all necessary supporting information, follow-up action should begin no later than 30 days from the date the claim was filed. Consideration should be given to initiating contact in less than 30 days if the normal turnaround time from insurance companies is 15 days or less, or if it is a large balance (Ibid.). Since the majority of revenue will be generated by insurance, time must not be wasted by extending the follow-up beyond 30 days. Contact with the insurance company should be initiated after 30 days have lapsed and no correspondence has been received.

It is important to ask when the claim will be processed and paid. Sometimes there is a difference between the processing time and the payment time. If the insurance company representative states that the claim or other required material has not been received, information should be obtained on exactly what is needed and specifically to whom it is to be sent. It is better to supply the requested information as soon as possible than to debate whether or not the information was previously sent and/or received.

Time should be saved at the end of each day to gather information on all claims for which insurance companies say additional information or billing is needed. Approximately 30 to 45 minutes should be enough time to gather this information and get it in the mail or use the fax machine to ensure timely receipt.

Once resolutions on claims have been achieved, an inquiry should be made about processing and payment procedures, and performance goals or objectives for processing and paying those claims.

Visits to Insurance Companies

In addition to the usual series of two or three tracer letters to the insurance companies, copies to patients on small balances, and telephone calls to insurance companies, one further step toward better communication needs to be taken. Managers should visit Blue Cross/Blue Shield and all insurance companies and/or commercial carriers that collectively represent 80 percent or more of their medical groups' cash flow (dollar volume).

There are several benefits to making personal visits. First, visits promote a better understanding of how each insurance company and employer operates. They make it easier to determine exactly what an insurance company looks for when processing claims. Second, face-to-face contact is established with people who would otherwise only be known over the telephone. This provides an opportunity for managers to show that they work for an honest and reputable medical group that provides quality care to its patients. Third, mutual problems that are causing payment delays can be discussed, opening the door to better rapport between the medical group and the insurance company.

Visits to insurance companies or employers may reveal that they have ineffective systems for processing claims and untrained personnel, or they may reveal that the problem lies with the medical group personnel. Only by seeing firsthand how claims are processed can a determination be made on what action must be taken to improve the process.

It is helpful to set up a file on all insurance carriers. The file should include names, addresses, and telephone numbers for each company, the employers they insure, and the names of claims managers. Details should also be obtained about claims processing procedures: time involved, paperwork, routing, how problems are handled, whether or not claims go through the employer, and more. What specific information does the insurance carrier look for — for example, exception criteria, length of stay, charges for a particular diagnosis, or dollar amount of ancillary charges? This information should be passed on to administrative personnel so decisions can be made on what to do when claims include charges that exceed the criteria.

Notes should be kept on reasons why claims are not paid. These should be reviewed with the billers and passed on to the registration staff and financial counselors. There may be specific steps to follow in order to provide billers with information that could help eliminate payment delays.

Getting Others Involved

If there is no response or cooperation from the insurance company, the next step is to call the patient or the employer of the patient. The patient should have received some type of letter prior to this point explaining that the claim has not been paid and that his or her assistance is requested. The facts need to be presented clearly, then the patient and the employer should be asked to call the insurance company to inquire about the status of the claim and why it has not yet been paid.

The patient should be provided with the telephone number, address, and name of the individual with whom medical group personnel have been corresponding. The patient should be informed that he or she is ultimately responsible for the bill, and if payment is not made within a specified period of time, the patient will have to pay (Ibid.).

Collecting from insurance carriers is the area where at least 80 percent of efforts should be concentrated in terms of telephone activity or follow-up. The balance of collection activities should be spent on self-pay billing and reimbursement; the group's computer system should be set up to provide notices and do most follow-up correspondence on small balances.

Managed Care Contracts

Managed care contracts — health maintenance organizations (HMOs) and preferred provider organizations (PPOs) — present unique problems due to their special requirements. A common obstacle is the need for precertifications or preauthorizations. These carriers also typically need specific claim forms that the patient must supply. Follow-up of claims often centers around receiving authorization for treatment prior to providing treatment. It is important to know the correct procedures and guidelines in applying for an appeal for coverage. This appeal process should begin as soon as any delay becomes apparent.

Most managed care contracts have a timely payment provision (usually 30 to 45 days). It is important to hold the HMO or PPO to the contract. One proven technique is to send an itemized listing of claims that are beyond the contractual payment guidelines. For each claim, the "violation of contract" should be indicated. This will get the attention of the HMO or PPO.

It is important to put extra pressure on the HMO or PPO because most managed care contracts do not allow collection from the patient. However, this does not mean the patient or employer cannot be contacted to let them know about any problems with getting payment from the HMO or PPO.

SUMMARY OF KEY STRATEGY 5

Most medical group practice cash flow comes from third parties. Therefore, this area deserves major attention. In developing a third-party recovery strategy, the following steps should be considered:

1. Train personnel to obtain needed data and facilitate billing procedures for all of the various insurance companies. Get it right initially. Stay on top of insurance company requirements.

2. Devise billing control forms to review data and to make adjustments when necessary.

3. Start telephone follow-up to insurance companies with larger balances at 15 to 30 days. Use letters on smaller balances only. Get the patient involved to help collect from the third party.

4. Be tougher on insurance companies than on debtors in the self-pay sector.

5. Research and know the insurance companies that make up the majority of insured patients' accounts receivable. Know what it takes to get those bills paid quickly.

6. When collection from the insurance company proves difficult, get the employee and/or employer involved. In cases of severe negligence, contact the state insurance commissioner's office.

7. Concentrate most collection follow-up in this area, for two reasons: it is where the majority of money is tied up, and it is generally the easiest to collect.

KEY STRATEGY 6:
REDUCE SELF-PAY CONTRACTS

An important aspect of improving cash flow in medical groups is getting someone else to finance most of the self-pay receivables. In other words, it is desirable to let financial institutions carry accounts that need monthly payments. Ideally, contract payments on large balances should be avoided by medical groups. They tie up cash, require collection follow-up, and generally are too costly to carry. Since charging interest has never been a viable alternative for health care receivables, finding an alternate method to handle self-pay accounts that require long-term monthly payments is in order. Credit cards and bank financing can provide this alternative.

Major Credit Cards

Most health care organizations honor major credit cards to settle current and past-due accounts. The majority of administrators and collection personnel feel this is a positive step toward more up-to-date reimbursement procedures.

If a survey were taken of patients today, how many would know that major credit cards are an acceptable payment option? Unless credit cards are being "sold" effectively, it is probably a lot fewer than generally imagined.

Using charge cards to get payment from patients is a proven way to increase collections. Many patients may not have cash to pay in full, but they do have credit cards available. All a medical group needs to do is make patients aware of the fact that credit cards are accepted for payment, then convince them that charging their bills is the right thing to do. The following tips have been proven effective:

- **Put signs up.** Signs need to be readily visible to the patient. Post them at entrances, the business office, cashier offices, and registration points — anywhere the patient can see them.

- **Put the credit card option on statements.** All statements should make it very clear that credit cards are accepted. Do not hide the information on the back of the statement. Also, make it very simple for the patients to put credit card information on the statement and send it back.

- **Include the information in the credit policy.** Make sure the medical group credit policy points out that credit cards can be used instead of cash. The more options patients have from which to choose, the more likely they are to pay in full.

- **"Sell" credit cards constantly.** Patients do not always pay attention to signs, statements, or credit policy. Cashiers and collectors must tell patients about the credit card option, and they must be trained to take charge payments.

- **Convince patients that charging is the right thing to do.** Many patients do not want to put medical bills on their credit cards because they feel charge cards are for "fun" things, or they do not want to pay interest. They will need to be convinced that paying now is the right thing to do.

  Try motivators such as, *"I understand your concern, but won't you feel better knowing you have paid the medical group that gave you excellent medical care?"* Or, *"Paying this bill in full now on your credit card means you won't have to worry about it anymore. You'll be able to make small monthly payments on your credit card instead of paying us with cash right now."*

- **Overcome excuses.** Patients will offer many excuses for not paying by credit card. Be prepared to overcome these excuses.

  "My credit card is to the limit." Ask questions. Find out what the limit is, the current balance, how long they have had the card, and if they have a good credit history. If they have had the card for over one year and have been current, it may be possible for them to increase their limit. Or, they may be able to charge at least a portion of the bill on the credit card, and set up arrangements for the balance.

  "I can't afford to put it on my credit card." It may be necessary to explain to patients that they owe the same amount regardless of whether or not it is on the credit card. Charging a bill does not increase the balance, although interest must be paid for the luxury of paying in monthly installments. The medical group does not offer this luxury.

Using credit cards has become a way of life for most Americans. However, many patients are not aware that health care providers take credit cards. Once patients are aware, and if credit cards are sold effectively, it will become natural for them to charge their medical bills, too.

Medical Credit Cards

In addition to the major credit cards available for payment, medical credit cards are attracting attention as another means of financing self-pay accounts. Medical credit card programs allow patients to apply for credit and maintain an open-ended, revolving charge card for use at medical facilities only.

The credit card company charges the patient interest on the unpaid balance and usually discounts the bill paid to the provider to cover the fee. A medical credit card program can be very effective for emergency care because the bill is usually relatively small, and the card is a ready solution for immediate payment.

Bank Financing

Bank financing is not a new tool to medical group administrators, but can still be an effective means to control, and even reduce, monthly outstanding balances. First, a local bank should be selected that is well known to area patients, and a loan program should be arranged that is easy for both the medical group and patients to handle. It is important to get a quote on competitive interest rates in order to make the repayment plan sellable. Since all notes will probably be endorsed with full recourse, it should be easy to persuade the bank to handle the program. The bank's procedures for advertising, collecting, and soliciting customers should be noted, as well as whether it is interested in new customers.

If the patient has little or no insurance and the account balance is over $100, the patient can sign a note. The monthly payment will then be made to the bank and not to the group practice. Having the account paid in this manner eliminates the need for additional billing and collection paper work, and the account is quickly cleared from the medical group records. In turn, the medical group is paid in full by the bank. With this arrangement, the monthly payment fits the patient budget; the bank draws interest on the account; and most important to the medical group, receivables are reduced.

When a patient agrees to sign a note, a bank credit application must be completed, including all of the patient's credit information: address, number of dependents, employer, position, length of employment, monthly income, where the patient banks, mortgage information, credit references, and other relevant facts. The patient must also sign a promissory note for the total of the principal plus interest. The note indicates the amount of the loan, the proceeds, the interest, and the number and amount of monthly installments. Notes should not be written for less than $100, nor should they be extended for more than three years. The bank remits to the medical group the proceeds of the note.

Usually, the bank will purchase all notes without prior credit checking and with no restrictions on the terms other than the established minimum amount and loan period. However, these notes are subject to full recourse, which means repurchase by the group practice if default on payment occurs. On loans that are not being properly paid, the bank will normally contact the patient by letter and one follow-up phone call when necessary. The medical group must repurchase the note before it is 90 days past due, or earlier if the bank deems it uncollectible. This might occur, for example, when the patient is unemployed or has filed bankruptcy.

The bank normally will not take legal action and usually does not engage in collection on loans of this type. If a patient makes no payment, the medical group must repurchase the note. Delinquent accounts that are repurchased should be sent to a collection agency without delay for the total amount (principal plus any accrued interest) to be paid.

This type of bank financing is ordinarily not solicited by a bank because of the size of the patients' notes and the marginal nature of the credit. It is offered only as an accommodation to the medical group whose account balance at the participating bank warrants this consideration.

Payment Monitoring Programs

Many collection agencies and outside vendors offer payment monitoring programs to handle long-term, contract accounts. These programs allow medical groups to remove self-pay contracts from the accounts receivable, and the agency then monitors the arrangements for a fee (8 to 10 percent contingency rate is normal).

This type of program should be used as a last resort, after all credit card or bank financing approaches have been exhausted, because payment in full will be delayed. However, payment monitoring programs should be used as a viable alternative to handling long-term arrangements within the medical group. The agency will usually do a better job of following up on delinquencies, plus the account can be transferred into the normal collection process quickly if the patient defaults. The collection fee would then increase to the usual rate.

SUMMARY OF KEY STRATEGY 6

When designing a policy to reduce or handle self-pay accounts, these ideas should be incorporated:

1.   It is best to stay away from carrying contract payments on large self-pay accounts. These balances need follow-up, and pull the medical group manager and staff away from more profitable accounts while inflating the outstanding accounts receivable.

2.   Utilizing credit cards improves cash flow and eliminates follow-up on this type of account in the self-pay category.

3.   Bank financing is another way of doing business today. Poor public relations should not be a concern. Patients will accept the concept easier than expected. Since most businesses and many hospitals are utilizing this type of repayment plan, there is no reason for medical groups to overlook this option as a means of improving cash flow.

4.   After all efforts for payment in full have been exhausted, a payment monitoring program at a local agency is preferable to handling long-term contracts within the medical group.

KEY STRATEGY 7:
DESIGN FORM LETTERS THAT WORK

Form letters and notices are not as effective for collecting health care dollars as they were years ago. Therefore, statements, letters, and notices generated by the computer must be constructed to pay off as much as possible.

Collection letters and notices can and should be used to some degree. Careful design is important to insure the best results, both in collection and public relations. Development should be geared towards obtaining payment in full and promoting faster paying habits, while maintaining favorable patient relations.

Why Patients Do Not Pay

When developing letters or notices, the five main reasons why a debtor does not pay should be kept in mind. It helps to take a moment to put oneself in the patient's place before putting thoughts on paper. These are the most common reasons for nonpayment:

- Temporary lack of funds
- Dissatisfaction
- Overlooked statements
- No intention of payment
- Belief that insurance will pay

With these in mind, five rules should be incorporated into letter and statement writing:

1) Assume the money will be paid. Be polite and positive.
2) Never imply an individual is dishonest.
3) Be firm, but courteous.
4) Show willingness to cooperate with the patient.
5) Advise if insurance has paid a portion of the statement — use names, dates, and amounts.

Collection Letters

Collection letters can be expensive and may not provide the desired results; therefore, they must not be relied on as a major part of the follow-up system. When collection letters are used, they should be short and to the point. Careful composition will help make them count. It is critical to consider them from the point of view of public relations as well as collections.

The following guidelines should be observed when writing collection letters:

1. Do not write long letters. They discourage the reader.

2. Avoid unnecessary words that confuse the reader.

3. Avoid using trite expressions such as "we failed to receive your payment," "I beg to remain," or "please favor us."

4. Request a definite amount of money at a definite time. Use judgment, and do not request the impossible.

5. Include payment options such as credit card or bank financing in letters.

6. Compose the letters personally using your best judgment.

7. Avoid "I" trouble, such as "I expect" or "I cannot continue to."

8. Refrain from using sarcasm. Be firm, but keep a personal touch.

9. Outline letters so the approach is direct and in sequence.

10. Avoid humor in letters unless it is used with tact and finesse. It often can be dangerous.

11. Be human. Use words that stand for human beings, like names of persons or personal pronouns (you, he, she, we).

12. Admit mistakes. Do not hide them behind meaningless words.

13. Do not overwhelm the reader by being too intense or emphatic.

14. Strive for a tone of expression that is friendly, with simple dignity.

15. Always start with a positive, "selling" opening. Do not upset or anger the debtor at the outset.

16. Use no more than four paragraphs. Keep sentences under 30 words.

17. Say it simply. The shorter word is preferable to the longer word.

18. Preserve the patient's dignity and self-respect. Nothing is gained by strong statements.

19. Start with a favorable intention, then proceed to the middle of the letter. State your case clearly, giving the reader a reason to pay.

20. Visualize talking to one person.

21. Remember that the goal is to get patients to do something willingly. They must be motivated.

22.   Provide a means of responding to the letter (telephone number and address). Encourage the patient to contact the medical group.

23.   Include a payment stub and a return envelope.

Those who have done a lot of collection letter writing say the debtor will usually react favorably to the appeals of fair play, doing what is right, and a reminder that the patient was not denied medical services in his or her time of need. In other words, it is important to foster a desire for cooperation on the part of the debtor. Just having a bill does not mean the patient can, wants to, or will ever make payment. Motivation, not brow-beating, is the key. These "reasons" may be helpful in motivating payment by patients:

- Prompt payment builds peace of mind.
- The patient can be helped out of financial trouble.
- Delay in payment could mean more costs.
- Payment will help the debtor keep a good reputation.
- A good credit record is a valuable asset.

FIGURE 7-1.
SAMPLE COLLECTION LETTERS

SAMPLE 1.

PATIENT NAME _______________________________
ACCOUNT NUMBER _______________________
BALANCE DUE _____________________________

Our records indicate that you owe _______________ on your account.

We are sure this is an oversight and we can expect payment to be mailed today. Thank you in advance for your payment.

Sincerely,

SAMPLE 2.

PATIENT NAME _______________________________
ACCOUNT NUMBER _______________________
BALANCE DUE _____________________________

We have not received payment on your past due account in the amount of __________.
When services were needed, the medical group did not hesitate to provide them to you.

It is only fair to pay the full amount immediately.

Sincerely,

SAMPLE 3.

PATIENT NAME _______________________________
ACCOUNT NUMBER ___________________________
BALANCE DUE _______________________________

Our records indicate that you have not paid despite previous requests.

A good credit record is a valuable asset. However, failure to pay _______________ within 5 days will seriously jeopardize your credit standing with the medical group. In addition, a continued delay in payment could bring more costs to your account.

Avoid further collection procedures and pay the full balance due now!

Sincerely,

SAMPLE 4.

FINAL NOTICE

PATIENT NAME _______________________________
ACCOUNT NUMBER ___________________________
BALANCE DUE _______________________________

Your balance of _______________ is seriously past due.

Pay the balance due within 5 days or we will send your account to a collection agency or attorney.

Sincerely,

SAMPLE 5.

PATIENT NAME _______________________________
ACCOUNT NUMBER _______________________________
BALANCE DUE _______________________________

Thank you for using the services of the medical group. Your amount due is shown above.

If you are waiting for your insurance to pay, please remember that the balance is due in full within 30 days of the original statement, regardless of insurance delays.

The medical group honors credit cards as payment options for our patients. Please call our office if you have any questions.

Sincerely,

SAMPLE 6.

PATIENT NAME _______________________________
ACCOUNT NUMBER _______________________________
BALANCE DUE _______________________________

Account balances are due in full within 30 days from the original statement unless other arrangements have been agreed to.

Please use the enclosed envelope to mail your payment in full today. If you would like this balance placed on your credit card, phone our office.

If you have any questions concerning your account, please contact us today.

Sincerely,

SAMPLE 7.

PATIENT NAME _______________________________
ACCOUNT NUMBER _______________________________
BALANCE DUE _______________________________

Your account is past due. Payment in full is due immediately. This delinquent account may affect your credit rating.

Please mail payment in full today, or contact our office. The medical group honors credit cards for your convenience.

Sincerely,

SAMPLE 8.

PATIENT NAME _______________________________
ACCOUNT NUMBER _______________________________
BALANCE DUE _______________________________

TEN DAY FINAL NOTICE

Your overdue account has been brought to my attention with the recommendation that it be placed with a professional collection agency.

Payment in full must be received in our office within 10 days.

This balance can be placed on your credit card by calling our office with your card information.

Sincerely,

Insurance Follow-Up Letters

For the most part, letters are not an effective collection tool to use with insurance companies. Telephone calls are a more productive means of follow-up. Most insurance personnel will not respond to letters immediately; sometimes they will not respond at all. A telephone call demands an immediate response. Time should not be wasted sending letters on large balances. Tracers or letters should be limited to smaller balance accounts.

FIGURE 7-2.
SAMPLE INSURANCE FOLLOW-UP LETTERS

SAMPLE 1.

COMMUNITY MEDICAL CENTER

PATIENT ________________________________
INSURED ________________________________
DATE OF SERVICE ________________________
BALANCE DUE ____________________________
POLICY NUMBER __________________________

The patient was at our office from ______________ to ______________. It has been more than two weeks since an assignment of benefits and a statement were mailed to you, but as yet we have not received payment on this account.

We would appreciate your advising us as to the present status of this claim.

Sincerely,

SAMPLE 2.

COMMUNITY MEDICAL CENTER

PATIENT ________________________________
INSURED ________________________________
DATE OF SERVICE ________________________
BALANCE DUE ____________________________
POLICY NUMBER __________________________

Our office has previously written you concerning the above unpaid claim upon which an assignment of interest was given to us by your insured.

It has been at least 30 days since we forwarded the necessary documents for this claim to be processed and paid. We must hear from you immediately as to why the payment has been delayed.

Sincerely,

SAMPLE 3.

COMMUNITY MEDICAL CENTER

PATIENT ____

INSURED ____

DATE OF SERVICE ________________________________

BALANCE DUE ____________________________________

POLICY NUMBER __________________________________

On _____________ we billed your insurance company but as yet we have not received payment for the above charges. It is our policy that if payment from the insurance company is not received within sixty (60) days from the date of billing, the entire balance must be considered the patient's responsibility.

We would appreciate your forwarding the amount due to our office within five days from the date of this letter.

Sincerely,

Finally, when designing collection letters, the following points should be kept in mind:

1. Collection letters are expensive and get less than acceptable results; therefore, they should not be relied upon as a major portion of the follow-up system.

2. Notices are more effective and less expensive, so form letters should be kept to a minimum.

3. If collection letters are used, they should be kept short. Careful composition will help make them count. It is important to regard collection letters from the viewpoint of public relations as well as collection.

4. Letters must be reviewed periodically for needed changes.

Collection Notices and Statements

Because of the large volume of small, outpatient balances, automated statements must be as effective as possible. Patients often complain that health care bills and statements are difficult to understand, confusing, or do not provide enough information. These tips will help in the design of effective, "patient friendly" notices or statements:

1. Keep collection notices and statements simple. Avoid unnecessary words or information that will confuse the reader.

2. Include all pertinent information regarding the account (date of service, balance, account number), without overloading the notice with data.

3. Include a return envelope to make it easy for the patient to send payment.

4. Be sure the statement clearly points out that the medical group accepts credit cards as a payment option. If possible, include a tear off section for the patient to write in credit card information.

5. Notices should be geared toward obtaining payment in full rather than payment arrangements.

6. As with collection letters, keep public relations in mind when designing statements or notices.

7. The messages on notices should clearly state the status of the patient's account.

Since it is desirable for notices, automated or manual, to have as much impact on collections as possible, a significant amount of quality time should be spent in their design. The phrasing of the appeal and the layout of the form can have a positive or negative effect. The goal is to collect without creating unnecessary telephone calls and poor public relations.

In order for notices to have the greatest effect, considerable care and research should be put into their construction. The wording and format should be designed to motivate the debtor into action. The wording should use appeals which either increase desire to pay or lower resistance to paying. However, no matter how well composed, the notice will have no effect unless it captures the debtor's attention.

No attention, no collection! The following points regarding the design of notices may be helpful for drawing more attention:

*   **Size**. Larger things get more attention than smaller ones. Making notices larger is one way to increase the attention they receive.

*   **Motion**. Motion attracts attention. Arrows, ellipses, or other symbols can be used to draw the eye toward the important elements of the notice.

*   **Isolation**. Objects standing alone command attention. Notices should be designed so they are not cluttered and portions of the text are suitably isolated.

*   **Color**. Color is related to attention. Colors toward the red end of the spectrum have higher attention-getting value. Therefore, oranges, reds, yellows, and pinks should be used when possible. Goldenrod is a good collection color. Blue, white, green, and black are less desirable.

*   **Legibility**. Typefaces with fairly heavy strokes will help ensure readability.

FIGURE 7-3.
SAMPLE STATEMENT CYCLES

SMALL BALANCE — SELF-PAY

Four reminder statements within 75 days.
Prelist with agency at 90 days.
Agency write-off at 120 days.

MESSAGE #1 — Day 15
The balance due is your responsibility. Please mail in full payment today.

MESSAGE #2 — Day 35
This balance is past due. Please pay promptly and avoid further action.

MESSAGE #3 — Day 55
This balance is past due. Protect your credit record and pay now.

MESSAGE #4 — Day 75
FINAL NOTICE: This account will be placed with our collection agency or attorney unless full payment is received in seven days.

SMALL BALANCE — INSURANCE

Balance should be transferred to self-pay automatically in the system at day 45. Then, four reminder statements to patients within 90 days, starting at 45 days.
Prelist with agency at 90 days from discharge.
Agency write-off at 120 days.

MESSAGE #1 — Day 45
No insurance payment received.
Please call your insurance company.

MESSAGE #2 — Day 60
Your insurance has not paid bill. Please pay amount within seven days.

MESSAGE #3 — Day 75
Past due insurance amount. Pay balance due now to avoid further action.

MESSAGE #4 — Day 90
FINAL NOTICE: Account will be placed with a collection agency or attorney unless full payment is received in seven days.

LARGE BALANCE — SELF-PAY

Four statements within 90 days. These statements are a minor collection tool.
Telephone contacts (at least four) are required prior to 90 days.

MESSAGE #1 — Day 21
The balance due is your responsibility. Please mail in full payment today.
(Call patient)

MESSAGE #2 — Day 42
This balance is past due. Protect your credit record and pay now.
(Call patient)

MESSAGE #3 — Day 63
The balance is past due. Pay promptly and avoid further action.
(Call patient)

MESSAGE #4 — Day 90
FINAL NOTICE: This account will be placed with our collection agency or attorney
unless full payment is received in seven days.
(Call patient)

LARGE BALANCE — INSURANCE

Four statements within 90 days. These statements are a minor collection tool.
Telephone contacts to the patient and insurance (at least four) are required prior to 90
days.

MESSAGE #1 — Day 30
No insurance payment received. Please call your insurance company.
(Call insurance)

MESSAGE #2 — Day 51
Your insurance has not paid. Please pay amount within seven days.
(Call insurance and patient)

MESSAGE #3 — Day 72
Past due insurance account. Pay balance due now to avoid further action.
(Call patient)

MESSAGE #4 — Day 90
FINAL NOTICE: Account will be placed with a collection agency or attorney unless full
payment is received in seven days.
(Call patient)

**SUMMARY OF
KEY STRATEGY 7**

When designing the total collection system, including collection letters and statements, it is important to keep these guidelines in mind:

1. If form letters will be used in follow-up, design them with care, keeping both collection and public relations in mind.

2. Remember that fewer form letters are better than more. Notices are more effective and less expensive.

3. Don't rely on collection letters and statements as major parts of the follow-up system, especially for large balances. Telephone calls will get better results.

4. Keep form letters and statements simple. Don't confuse the reader.

5. Review form letters and notices at least once per year for necessary changes.

KEY STRATEGY 8:
EXPAND DATA PROCESSING PAYOFF

Data processing has become such a major tool for collection management in medical groups that an entire book could be devoted to this aspect of controlling receivables. Three major aspects of data processing that have a significant effect on collections will be highlighted here:

1. Accuracy
2. Exception reporting
3. Effective use of statements

Guidelines for Management

These general guidelines for managing a data processing system deserve special attention:

1. **Get to know the patient accounting software.** Most patient accounting software is equipped with a number of standard daily, weekly, and monthly reports. For the reports to be useful, it is important for the manager to be aware of data selection criteria, sorting parameters, and any usual data processing posting cycles or interface limitations. Time invested in exploring the basics of a system will be more than offset by a new sense of the software's capabilities (and limitations).

2. **Become computer literate.** While it is not necessary for the manager to be a programmer or systems analyst, a basic understanding of computer terms and concepts is essential. This understanding will make it possible to explain needs in terms that a data processing professional can understand.

3. **Define what needs to be reviewed.** Reports that help manage accounts receivable are not necessarily the same ones that are valuable in the collection process. Aging criteria for control reports should be based on discharge date. Collection tools are generally based on last activity date. It is important not to make the mistake of believing these are the same thing.

4. **Keep reports simple.** The more complex the design of selection and sort criteria, the greater the potential for creating a "black hole;" that is, a group of accounts that inadvertently do not meet any of the conditions that have been set, and therefore are not worked or controlled on a timely basis.

5. **Talk to staff and make adjustments as needed.** Reports designed a year ago may not have any value today. Selection criteria, sort parameters, and billing cycles need to be reviewed and revised on a regular basis. Staff members should be asked how they use computer reports and why they are not used (if that is the case), as well as what could be done to improve their value.

Accuracy of Aged Trial Balance

Computer printouts may reflect certain types of inaccuracies on individual accounts, but the most common type of inaccuracy seems to be a patient liability incorrectly appearing as an insurance liability or vice versa. If aged trial balances (ATBs) are analyzed with incorrect dollar totals, reviews and actions may be inappropriate and could lead to public relations problems.

An incorrectly placed balance will normally show up in the area of insurance. This is because most medical groups have some policy regarding the length of time that accounts will be deemed the insurance company's responsibility before they are considered the patient's liability. For example, if a carrier does not pay within 45 days of billing, an attempt may be made to collect from the patient involved and let him or her handle the insurance company.

When a medical group has such a policy, this question should be asked: "Is the policy being carried into computer programs?" If not, data processing personnel must be consulted to define the terms of the policy and to write and implement programs to put the policy into effect.

Exception Reporting

Providing data for decisions through exception reporting is probably the most effective tool any computer can furnish a manager. Computers store and print vast amounts of raw data. However, data becomes useful information only after it has been encapsulated and interpreted. Concise, up-to-date information continues to be increasingly important in the area of accounts receivable where the size of the file makes it difficult to review account by account.

Any computerized accounts receivable file should have report selection capabilities available. This means it should be possible to look at an abbreviated file listing where the printed accounts satisfy one or a number of specific parameters. Data processing personnel should be able to provide management with a selected report based on virtually any data elements contained in the receivables file. For example, it may be desirable to look only at self-pay accounts which have had no payment posted for the last 60 days.

In addition to selected reporting, encapsulated management reports should also be available. A typical management report sent to the credit manager could be a one- or two-page synopsis of unsettled accounts receivable and number of days outstanding for all categories of payment. Such a report would normally be run on a monthly basis and would be useful in determining trends in receivables and potential problem areas. It can also be used as a reporting tool by the manager. This would eliminate any transcription or retyping by staff in reporting to the next level of administration.

Outlined below are selected exception reports from data processing systems that may be helpful in analyzing receivables.

High-to-low balance by payment category. This report includes accounts with the highest balances within self-pay, Blue Cross/Blue Shield, third party, Medicare, Medicaid, worker's compensation, and so on.

Insurance payments. This system can be used to monitor the payment activity of any insurance company that provides coverage to patients. Each insurance company handled through this system is identified by special open claims information with the insurance company's name, address, and telephone number.

Patient balances per category. With this report, several balances incurred by a patient or a family of patients can be included on a single printout. The entry of a category code would indicate the type of balance on each transaction. This capability is very useful if there are patients who keep multiple balances open at the same time. For example, a patient may have an open Medicaid balance that is distinct from current charges which are the patient's responsibility. This allows keeping balances separate but associated with the same account number. There are several significant benefits to this method:

- Several account records do not have to be established for the same account record in the database. There is no duplication of account information.

- All account information for all balances can be accessed at the same time. It is evident when an account has several balances, and how much is owed on each of those balances.

- Each balance can be handled individually in terms of statements, insurance, and other reports. For example, it can be specified that all self-pay statements are to be mailed, but all Medicaid statements suppressed. One or more insurance companies' payments can be directed to the appropriate type of balance.

- All accounts receivable reports reflect the correct amounts per category code.

- All reporting documents reflect amounts separated by a category code, even though there may be several balances on one account record.

Credit manager's exception list. This report provides a listing of all patients who have appointments in the next "x" days and who have been flagged as having unacceptable credit status. The flagging is done through the system using a specified amount and time parameters.

Credit balances. All credit balances, even those only two weeks old, are shown.

Unpaid third-party accounts. A listing is provided of all accounts over 30 days from billing. Note: the time frame is an arbitrary figure; 45 days, 15 days, or another length of time may be preferred.

Self-pay accounts with no payments. A listing is provided of all self-pay accounts with no payment listed for at least 60 days. Once again, the time frame is an arbitrary figure; the time parameter should be selected to fit group needs.

Collector performance. This report reflects the overall effectiveness of each collector. It may also be compiled per biller or cashier. A sample is provided in *Figure 8-1*.

Comparison of collections to goal. A compilation is made of total daily collections for the current month compared to set goals. A sample is provided in *Figure 8-2*.

Collection agency performance. This report shows the collection agency's current and year-to-date collections and the total amount of possible collection balance pending. A sample is provided in *Figure 8-3*.

Aged trial balance by collection agency. The aging of accounts listed for collection by date of listing is shown.

Unpaid accounts submitted to collection agency. This report reflects all accounts submitted to a collection agency prior to 90 days and showing no subsequent payment. The time frame is an arbitrary period; it may be valuable to review several such reports varying the time limit.

Dollars collected at time of service. An ongoing account is provided of payments received at time of service.

Statements sent to the patient. All accounts are listed which have received, for example, at least four statements.

Grouping by category. This selection is particularly valuable when used in combination with age of account or number of statements sent. It is also important that computer printouts display the date of preparation of the last statement and highlight accounts for which no statement has ever been prepared. Most computer systems allow for the inhibition of statements under certain circumstances. Detailing these accounts will allow for internal collection analysis.

Aged trial balance arranged by guarantor or responsible party. Such a report is arranged alphabetically by guarantor with all the accounts for which the patient is responsible listed after his or her name. This will assist the credit personnel in telephone follow-up since all of the accounts can be referenced in the same call. For this purpose, guarantor's address and telephone number should be displayed on the report as well.

This report is also useful for posting cash. When a check is received from the guarantor, the cashier can easily determine the account(s) to which the check should be applied. Similarly, if the guarantor has a credit balance account, that credit can be easily posted against another outstanding balance.

Self-pay contracts. For those medical groups writing contracts with self-pay patients, a report of delinquent contract accounts should be available. If received on a weekly basis, this report should be relatively short, allowing for follow-up.

FIGURE 8-1.
COLLECTOR PERFORMANCE REPORT

RUN DATE 6/ /92   03 JOHN DOE   PAGE 3

| L.OB | CURRENT | | | | | YEAR TO DATE | | | | | AVG MONTHLY |
NO.	LISTINGS	ACCTS	AVERAGE	COLLECTIONS	%	LISTINGS	ACCTS	AVERAGE	COLLECTIONS	%	LISTINGS
0001	.00		.00	.00	.0	108.00	1	108.00	.00	.0	1 .50
0002	.00		.00	.00	.0	669.75	2	334.88	.00	.0	8 .72
0003	7,050.01	8	881.25	6,023.95	85.4	389,368.60	690	564.30	48,195.25	12.4	48,671.03
0004	18,238.93	152	119.99	1,737.39	9.5	48,047.28	328	146.49	18,293.93	38.1	6,005.91
0005	131,479.21	203	647.68	18,529.03	14.1	816,185.79	1,470	555.23	136,963.69	16.8	102,023.22
0006	212,952.71	1,003	212.32	94,474.89	44.4	1,013,966.19	4,336	233.85	594,420.28	58.6	126,745.77
0008	.00		.00	.00	.0	164,513.17	685	240.17	139,923.81	85.1	20,564.15
0012	17.00	1	17.00	17.00	100.0	12,466.07	43	289.91	4,900.25	39.3	1,558.26
0013	.00		.00	.00	.0	.00		.00	657.42	39.3	.00
COLLECTOR TOTALS											
	369,737.86	1,367	270.47	120,782.26	32.7	2,445,324.85	7,555	323.67	943,354.63	38.6	305,665.61

FIGURE 8-2.
REPORT COMPARING COLLECTIONS TO GOAL

GOAL TO ACTUAL REPORT　　　　06/01/92

COLLECTOR	DAILY GOAL	DAILY COLL	%	MONTH GOAL	MTD COLL	%
07		4,303.25			37,725.55	
91		.00			.00	
TOTALS	3,250.00	4,303.25	132.41	65,000.00	37,725.55	58.04
01		306.00			3,405.15	
02		.00			.00	
TOTALS	750.00	306.00	40.80	15,000.00	3,405.15	22.70
01		935.00			18,332.04	
02		.00			29,081.75	
09		2,560.81			3,156.87	
10		.00			109.10	
12		.00			1,243.18	
70		.00			.00	
71		.00			4,746.75	
TOTALS	6,250.00	3,495.81	55.93	125,000.00	56,669.69	45.34
03		.00			68,386.05	
07		.00			.00	
13		.00			.00	
90		.00			20.00	
91		.00			.00	
93		.00			448.32	
95		.00			4,784.43	
96		.00			10.00	
97		.00			355.66	
TOTALS	6,000.00	.00	.00	120,000.00	74,004.46	61.67
RECOVERY TOTALS	16,250.00	8,105.06	49.88	325,000.00	171,804.85	52.86
˙DELINQUENT PREMIUMS		.00			47,724.30	

˙NOT IN GOAL OR TOTALS

FIGURE 8-3.
COLLECTION AGENCY PERFORMANCE REPORT

RUN DATE 6/1/82   PAGE 19

L.OB NO.	CURRENT					YEAR TO DATE					AVG MONTHLY
	LISTINGS	ACCTS	AVERAGE	COLLECTIONS	%	LISTINGS	ACCTS	AVERAGE	COLLECTIONS	%	LISTINGS
0003	.00		.00	255.58	118.1	3,730.74	19	196.35	359.58	9.6	466.34
0004	23.50CR	1	23.50CR	307.21	307.3	2,029.60	5	405.92	1,034.61	51.0	253.70
0005	5,013.45	3	1,671.15	340.00	6.8	48,328.38	54	894.97	8,973.18	18.6	6,041.05
0006	6,528.00	5	1,305.60	323.05	4.9	18,001.09	55	327.29	9,241.82	51.3	2,250.14
COLLECTOR TOTALS	11,517.95	9	1,279.77	1,225.84	10.6	72,089.81	133	542.03	19,609.19	27.2	9,011.23

Counselor accounts. If the patient counselor system is used to assign responsibility of accounts, each counselor should have a separate balance report defining only his or her accounts. This technique reduces the bulk of the individual reports and serves as a management tool for measuring each counselor's collection effectiveness.

Summary analysis. Finally, the administrator or manager should have available upon request a summarized analysis of receivables. This report shows the dollars and, if appropriate, the number of accounts involved monthly in each major category. A report of revenue figures by category should be maintained to allow for easy calculation of outstanding days per primary payer, which is an important factor in determining where to devote the greatest collection efforts.

Effective Use of Statements

One of the routine jobs eliminated by computerization of receivables is the manual preparation of statements, notices, and letters. In many cases, the medical group prints statements, but does not exercise adequate control over the frequency, sorting, color, wording, and overall impact. The following areas should be considered:

1. **Are zero balance statements printed?** If they are, the computer can suppress the printing and save the cost of forms.

2. **Are credit balance statements mailed?** In most cases, these are used as a review tool for possible refunds or location of incorrectly posted payments. Two alternatives might be considered here. Either the statements could be computer sorted so such statements can all be directed to the attention of one person, or the computer could prepare a separate list of credit balance accounts.

3. **How are special collection messages handled?** Proper use of color and wording will increase collections with these statements.

4. **Has the data mailer or envelope concept been considered?** This is a computer-printed form which contains a return envelope and is immediately ready for mailing. Manual sorting, stuffing, and postage metering are eliminated, which can add one or two days to total outstanding days.

5. **Is automatic rollover of insurance billing to self-pay accounts used where feasible?**

6. **Do automatic statements get special attention?** Proper color, cycling, and wording will increase collections, decrease number of outstanding accounts, and free staff to concentrate on collecting large balance accounts. Key Strategy 3 and Key Strategy 7 provide more information on letter and notice design.

**SUMMARY OF
KEY STRATEGY 8**

The computer can be one of the accounts receivable manager's greatest assets by:

1.   Ensuring input data is accurate. Faulty information makes for poor decisions.

2.   Providing sophisticated and creative exception reporting.

3.   Maximizing the impact of statements and claim forms through proper design and mailing schedules.

KEY STRATEGY 9:
ANALYZE TO GET THE
"BIGGEST BANG FOR THE BUCK"

Too often, when the administrator says to the accounts receivable manager, "Get the receivables down" or "Improve the cash flow," the manager is frustrated and confused as to how to improve the situation and where to begin in order to make an immediate and significant difference. Calling together the collection staff and asking them to collect more money leaves them just as frustrated as the accounts receivable manager, and seldom produces the kind of results that will substantially improve the medical group's financial situation. Experienced accounts receivable managers know that a great deal of time can be spent collecting accounts that do not make sizable reductions in the accounts receivable or notable increases in monthly collection totals.

Zeroing in on Major Problems

Analyzing accounts receivable, collection activities, debtors, and third-party payers can be helpful in zeroing in on major problems. It may point out specific areas where collection efforts are likely to get significant results.

Each time a patient account manager examines the group's data reports, new problems may be found. These problems may not be altogether new, but simply an outgrowth of another problem. Maybe a new procedure is causing a problem, or possibly an old problem is compounding itself and spreading to other areas. At any rate, the patient account manager is responsible for locating the source of the problem and for devising a solution to deal with it. However, before a solution can be initiated, the root of the problem must first be identified. In *Figure 9-1*, a flowchart is provided which depicts the development of problem identification and considerations for solutions.

The analyses mentioned here are just a few of the types that can be useful in determining where time and effort need to be spent in order to obtain the greatest collection results. They can also assist in confirming staff strengths and weaknesses, as well as identifying procedural problems or policy loopholes. These occurrences should be noted as results are analyzed:

* Illogical groupings of functions of staff members
* Turnover of accounts receivable and account aging trends
* Follow-up and turnover of large balance accounts
* Unusual write-offs
* Processing delays

FIGURE 9-1.
FLOWCHART OF PROBLEM IDENTIFICATION

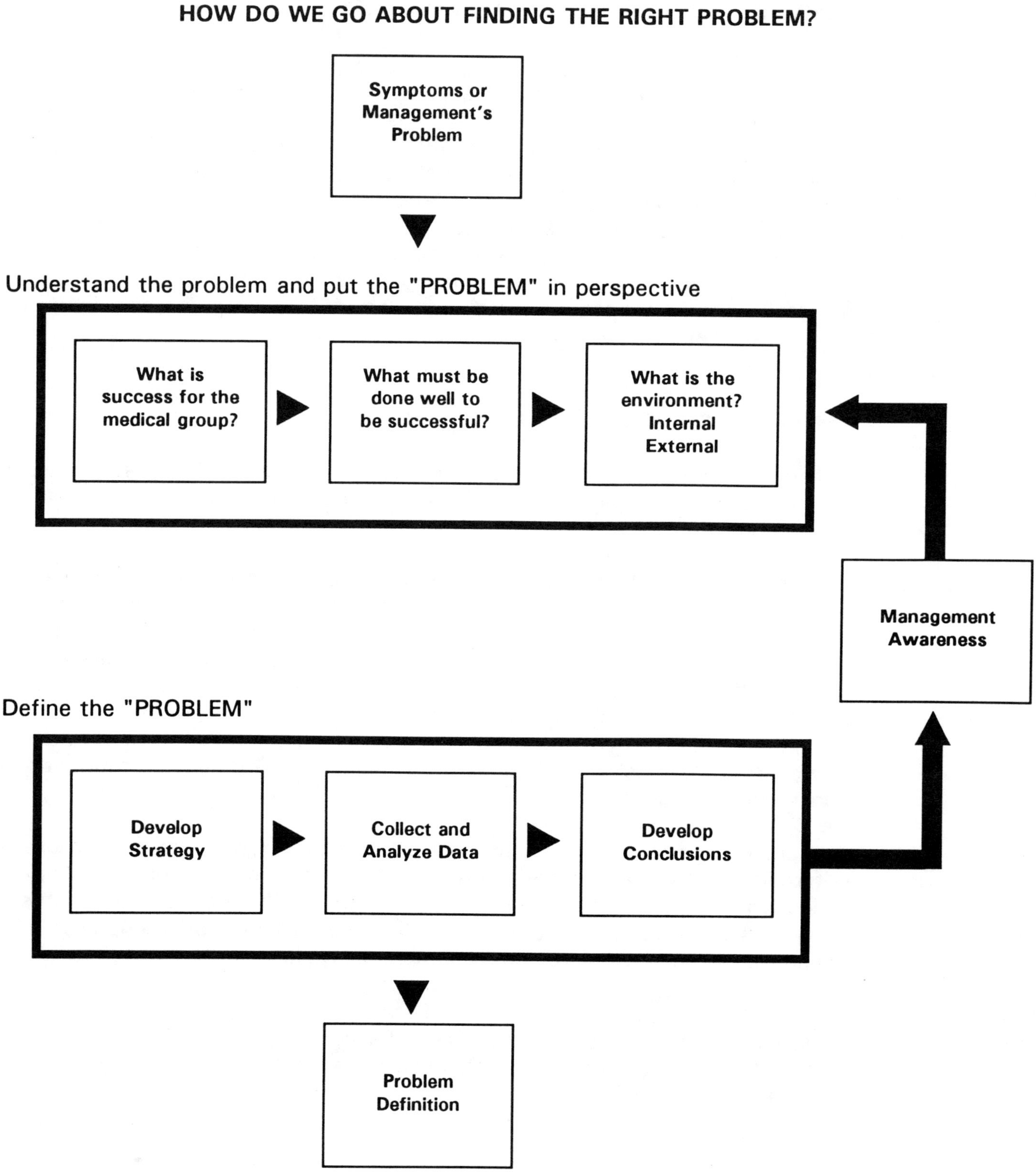

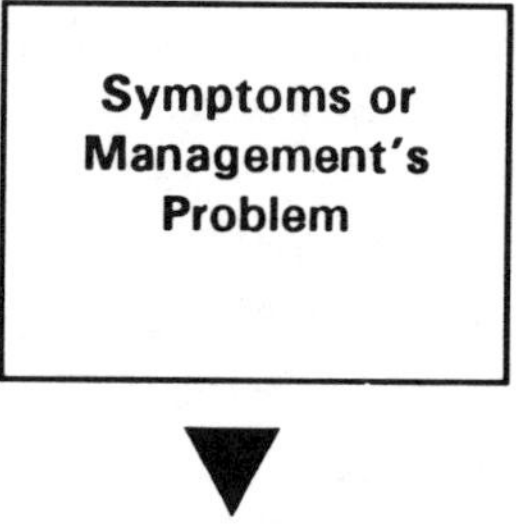

Payment History Analysis

One method of zeroing in on problem collection areas is to perform a payment history analysis. This is a relatively simple technique that does not take a lot of time, but gives direction to collection efforts and can produce results that may improve cash flow in a relatively short period of time.

The idea is to make an analysis of payment patterns within major areas that make up the accounts receivable. For instance, a payment history analysis can be made of Blue Cross/Blue Shield, Medicare, Medicaid, self-pay, and other categories within the medical group's total cash-flow picture. After analyzing the payment history of the major areas of outstanding accounts, a much clearer picture emerges of what needs to be done to increase collection totals and where to concentrate the greatest collection effort.

The analysis may bring out surprises: billings not promptly sent out from the billing department, improper collection activities and lax follow-up methods on Medicare accounts, two or three commercial insurance companies holding up most of the money in that category, accounts being sent to a collection agency without some prior collection effort, or poor collection procedures at time of service. Some of the problems may be outside the department, others may be inside. For instance, poor staffing, uneven work flow, and procedures not followed or updated may be hurting overall collections.

In any case, analysis enables the medical group administrator to evaluate the total outstanding receivables and the current collection system. After analysis, the administrator can concentrate on solving a particular problem in order to bring the quickest results — for example, clearing up a backlog of billing, adding staff to needed areas, collecting at the time of service, getting action from third parties, or decreasing the time an account is held before collection starts.

Sample payment histories with headings showing the kinds of information necessary to make a thorough analysis are provided in *Figure 9-2*, *Figure 9-3*, and *Figure 9-4*.

Developing Goals from Analysis

Collection goals can also be developed from analysis, new standards can be set, and a general method of approach can be put together for the entire accounts receivable staff after the manager has completed the analysis. A review of the accounts written off as bad debt or submitted to collection agencies can also be done after the account analysis. This will keep records up-to-date and of manageable size. After a staff member has completed the forms and filled in all columns from the actual account analysis, and the review of bad debt or accounts submitted to collection agencies has been completed, the manager can draw conclusions to assist in the development of a plan of action.

FIGURE 9-2.

PAYMENT HISTORY OF INSURANCE COMPANIES WITH MORE THAN ONE OCCASION

Insurance Company	No. of Billings	Total Days It Took to Pay per Each Bill	Average Days before Payment
Company A	5	14,89,67,7,36	43
Company B	4	11,2,26,14	13
Company C	3	10,13,28	17

SUMMARY:
Total average number of days from billing to payment: 26 days
Percent of patients who paid their share at time of service: 31%

FIGURE 9-3.

PAYMENT HISTORY ANALYSIS PER PATIENT

Patient Number	Service Date	Insurance Company	Date Insurance Billed	First Date Insurance Paid	Date Patient Paid	Amount Patient Paid at Service	Patient's Portion at Service	Insurance Portion	Total Bill
319250-40	03-16-80	Company A	03-27-80(11)	04-20-80(23)	03-16-80	$2.50	$2.50	$690.92	$693.42
322613-10	03-29-80	Company B	04-10-80(12)	04-21-80(11)	03-29-80	6.00	6.00	657.39	663.39
320946-60	02-07-80	Company C	02-22-80(15)	03-30-80(36)			14.50	919.49	933.99
322372-80	03-19-80	Company D	03-20-80(1)	04-24-80(35)	03-19-80	8.00	8.00	537.13	545.13

SUMMARY:

Average number of days from service to billing: 10 days

Average number of days from billing to payment: 27 days

Percent/total of patients' portions collected at time of service: 53%

Percent/patients who paid their portions in full at time of service: 90%

FIGURE 9-4.
HISTORY ANALYSIS OF WRITE-OFFS TO AGENCIES

Patient Number	Last Service Date	Phone Calls before Sending to Agency	Date Sent to Collection Agency	Months from Service to Turnover	Dollar Amount Submitted	Gross Amount Collected
322907-60	04-04-80	3	07-27-80	3.8	$ 16.00	$16.00
320467-30	01-21-80	9	05-31-80	4.3	492.83	300.00
322674-30	03-29-80	4	07-27-80	4.0	14.00	14.00
323145-30	04-13-80	8	07-27-80	3.5	264.96	264.96

SUMMARY:*

Average months from service to write-off:	4.0
Average number of phone calls before going to agency:	6.0
Percent gross dollar collected by agency:	76%

OBSERVATION: Spending more collection effort on accounts internally prior to forwarding them to a collection agency helps keep write-offs down while the percentage of accounts the agency collects remains the same.

*NOTE: These tabulations are based on only the four items listed in this figure.

Third-Party and Debtor Profile Analyses

Another type of analysis is the third-party profile. A sample third-party profile analysis form is provided in *Worksheet 4* in Appendix A. This analysis can be completed as delinquent insurance accounts are collected. Profiles assist the collector or administrator in identifying areas that need attention, particularly those related to third-party payers, where most money is collected and where most reimbursement time and effort should be concentrated. The third-party profile analysis will provide data and information which will help in the following areas:

- Identification of insurance companies that become collection problems
- Identification of reasons given by the third party for not paying
- Development of a third-party analysis fact sheet

This analysis, in turn, will help in collection from third-party payers by providing helpful "inside" information. A sample third-party analysis fact sheet is provided in *Worksheet 5* in Appendix A.

The debtor profile is an analysis similar to the third-party profile. This profile can be developed while the account is being collected by phone. After a sampling has been obtained, a profile of the debtor can be drawn to assist in collecting self-pay accounts. A sample self-pay debtor profile is provided in *Worksheet 6* in Appendix A.

Determining Individual Analytical Needs

It is only through investigation that the patient accounts manager or administrator is able to determine which analyses are appropriate for a medical group practice. Problems specific to a medical group because of location, patient demographics, type of group (health maintenance organization, preferred provider organization, fee-for-service group, etc.), participation in government reimbursement programs, specialty, and/or ancillary services may not be of concern to another group. Therefore, no two groups' analytical needs will ever perfectly match.

Also, because problems are perceived, defined, and finally solved, every medical group's analytical needs should fluctuate according to the priorities at any given time. Ideally, as a problem is identified and addressed, the patient accounts manager will choose to discontinue one type of analysis and initiate another. An accounts receivable analysis can help in sorting through problems and devising a plan to meet a group's particular analytical needs. A sample accounts receivable analysis worksheet is provided in *Worksheet 7* in Appendix A.

SUMMARY OF KEY STRATEGY 9

Time is well spent developing a continuing accounts receivable system of analysis that:

1. Will help in making decisions and make it possible to get "the biggest bang for the buck."

2. Will point out areas that need attention, including staff strengths and weaknesses, procedural and policy loopholes, and major problem areas.

3. Is done frequently enough to provide results, but does not tie up the manager or staff with constant projects that allow no time for action.

4. Will provide numerous perspectives of reported data to widen the conception of overall operations.

KEY STRATEGY 10: BUILD GOOD PUBLIC RELATIONS

Collections are, of course, the major function of the accounts receivable department. However, collections without favorable public relations will lead to the downfall of the person responsible and will collect fewer dollars in the long run. Building a collection system consistent with good public relations is critical to the success of a collection program.

The Customers

Health care is a service-oriented business. Patients, or customers, will judge the quality of a medical group practice based on the quality of customer service they receive. Staff in all areas of the medical group — from registration through collection — must be prepared to provide superior levels of service to each and every patient.

Most patients know little about clinical medicine, but they know a lot about how they like to be treated. If they are treated poorly during their visit to a facility, will they respond quickly and cooperate with payment? Probably not.

An accounts receivable manager *must* build public relations into the collection strategy and must train all staff members, from the receptionist through collection follow-up personnel, on collection techniques consistent with favorable patient relations. How well this is done will determine the success of the collection program.

The Manager

One administrator, when asked to name the desirable characteristics of a patient accounts manager, listed the following:

- Good communicator
- Good listener
- Tolerant and patient
- Good organizer
- Prompt in dealing with the patient by telephone or in person
- Good supervisor

The qualities stressed in this list are basically public relations characteristics. Nothing was mentioned about the ability to turn over cash flow expediently; perhaps this was to be understood. Public relations are an essential aspect of managing receivables. In fact, this may be the single most important aspect of collections to consider. Managers who have not mastered public relations skills, or do not give them proper emphasis, eventually move on to other fields — by request or otherwise.

Collection Policy, Procedures, and Practices

Maintaining favorable public relations while pursuing an active collection program does not depend entirely on favorable face-to-face or telephone contacts. There are other factors that determine favorable or unfavorable public relations. These include collection policy, procedures, practices, notices, and letters. Lack of attention to any one or all of these areas can cause adverse public relations in the collection process, no matter how skilled a staff may be at personal human relations.

A collection policy should stress maintaining the highest level of patient public relations while protecting receivables. It is important to develop a collection policy that covers the majority of situations that arise. This should be reviewed by the administration for approval and backing. When no collection policy exists, there is nothing to fall back on or refer to when a difficult public relations situation comes up. A policy provides backing, support, and direction for all staff.

After a collection policy has been developed and approved, the staff must be trained. Later, it is important to review the policy with staff from time to time, to be sure it is being followed. A lack of policy will come back to haunt a medical group time and again in the collection process.

Outdated procedures cause poor public relations. Existing collection procedures must be reviewed both before and after public relations problems come up. A questioning posture should be maintained: Does an existing procedure need to be revised? How will development of a new collection procedure affect public relations?

Another aspect of procedures that often leads to problems is staff failure to follow guidelines. Staff should be trained in the use of collection procedures and checked often enough to ensure procedures are being followed. Also, including staff in the development of procedures leads to a greater likelihood that procedures will be followed. *Figure 10-1* provides a list of collection practices to ensure good public relations in a collection program.

Collection Notices and Letters

In addition to collection policies, procedures, and practices, collection notices and letters also play an important role in determining favorable or unfavorable public relations. All notices and letters should be geared toward obtaining payment in full while preserving the patient's dignity and respect. Dunning notices designed to promote favorable relations will go a long way in improving a collection system.

FIGURE 10-1.
COLLECTION CODE OF ETHICS

1. Medical groups should explain fully to their patients the terms of any collection transaction.

2. Bills should be sent as soon as possible after the billing cycle ends — at least two weeks before the next payment is due.

3. Calls or correspondence from a patient claiming an error in billing should be acknowledged promptly.

4. Collection practices should be based on the presumption that every debtor intends to pay or would pay if able.

5. Late charges should be assessed only to the extent necessary to recover overall expenses caused by the delinquency.

6. Patient complaints concerning collection practices should be investigated immediately.

7. Collectors should be instructed to attempt to determine the cause of a delinquency and to indicate willingness to arrange a mutually satisfactory repayment schedule when appropriate.

8. Patients who show a sincere desire to repay their debts should be offered, if necessary, extended payment schedules, financing arrangements, or similar methods that would help re-establish solvency.

9. If the patient does not respond to an offer to help make alternative arrangements, the collector should explain the seriousness of continuing delinquency and advise the patient regarding courses of action.

10. While collectors have an obligation to honestly disclose to debtors and endorsees the remedies that may be invoked against them, legal action should not be cited unless it can and will be used.

11. Telephone calls should be placed between the hours of 8 A.M. and 9 P.M. in the patient's time zone, unless other times are more convenient for the patient.

12. Outside collection agencies, attorneys, process servers, and other agents employed to collect delinquent accounts should be furnished with written instructions on how patients are to be approached and which practices are and are not sanctioned.

13. Medical groups should be particularly careful in handling delinquencies due to a patient's dissatisfaction with services.

14. A patient's medical complaint, as a reason for not paying, should be referred immediately to the patient's physician for reconciliation.

The most effective collection methods are examined in an article published by the *Wisconsin Medical Credit Association.* A "soft letter" actually outcollects a "hard letter" almost two to one, according to a survey on collection letters for overdue accounts conducted over a reasonable period of time.

In *Writing Communications*, Robert Hay discusses a survey taken in a large department store's credit department. "Goodwill" letters outcollect "more direct, harder, firmer" collection letters by a substantial margin.

Scoring Public Relations Points

Many opportunities to score public relations points arise in a medical group setting. On the other hand, any employee who deals with the public presents the possibility of upsetting or alienating a patient. To better the chances of a positive patient encounter, the following customer relations principles should be incorporated into all dealings with patients:

- **Smile pleasantly.** Smiles are infectious. Even when speaking on the phone, a smile will come through.

- **Avoid terms of endearment.** Call the patient by his or her last name, using Mr., Mrs., or Ms. as a sign of respect.

- **Communicate effectively.** Be natural. Use words patients can understand. Be careful of technical jargon that may be unfamiliar to patients.

- **Look professional.** Adhere to dress codes. Look neat and clean.

- **Act professionally.** Avoid unprofessional mannerisms or slang. Never yell or make a scene in front of a patient or in a patient contact area.

- **Nonverbal communication.** Maintain eye contact. Watch posture and facial expressions.

- **Be perceptive.** Anticipate the patient's needs and respond. Be aware of common questions and concerns of patients and cater to them.

- **Handle complaints.** Do not become part of the problem. Let the patient calm down and address his or her concerns immediately. Remember, the patient probably will not pay until the complaint is resolved.

- **Respect the patient's dignity.** All patients deserve respect. Never say or do anything that may embarrass a patient.

- **Be patient.** Many patients are elderly or sick. Consider how you would want to be treated if in their place.

The Business Office

The importance of public relations in the business office of the medical group is often underestimated, in spite of the fact that this is where a great many public contacts are made. There are tales of red tape and endless forms to be filled out by the patient, and stories of office and collection personnel's indifference to patients entering or leaving the medical group. These may be exaggerations, yet health care providers are guilty to some degree.

The business manager cannot expect personnel in contact areas to naturally possess the correct attitudes and techniques for dealing with the public. It is the manager's responsibility to instruct these employees in the importance of patient relations.

A Public Relations Training Program

All office personnel should be briefed in the broad purposes of the medical group. Employees need general knowledge of practice operations and how they are supported. They should learn where patients' money goes when bills are paid, why costs are rising, and what kind of advance medical care the group offers. Employees who are up to date on this information can pass it along to the patients or public whenever necessary.

Cross-training on all functions within the business office will increase employee knowledge, thus providing the opportunity to respond promptly and accurately to patient concerns. A basic knowledge of psychology is also useful, since human nature is as much a source of difficulty as are financial problems in bill collection.

A training program on human relations can significantly improve public relations in the business office. This includes practicing specific techniques to improve how staff responds to patients. Tape-recorded examples of personal contacts with patients and actual role playing by members of the class can be incorporated into the program. After all, an awareness of the importance of strong public relations is worthless if the techniques are not carried out by the employees involved in the collection process.

Frequent training sessions and patient relations reminders are essential to providing favorable patient relations as the entire staff will be educated on why good human relations are important to group operations and cash flow.

Fielding Complaints

Why are strong public relations so important in the collection of health care accounts — more so than in any other type of credit? Extremely poor press fosters the public's adversity toward medical charges. Consequently, it does not take much to spark a fire, and "fires" slow down collection.

Administrators are particularly sensitive to complaints involving charges and collection procedures. They simply do not like to field complaints in this area. One way to combat complaints to administration is to intercept calls before they get there. This can be accomplished by developing a system where the administrator's secretary will intercept calls and forward the complaints to the patient accounts manager for resolution. The manager must in turn supply the administrator with proof the complaint was resolved within a 24-hour period, if possible. A form can be used to communicate what action was taken by the manager to appease the patient. Administration then has the option to follow up, if the situation warrants further action. A sample patient complaint form is provided in *Figure 10-2*. Most administrators will admit openly that they dislike fielding patient complaints and should respond well to this process.

FIGURE 10-2.
PATIENT COMPLAINT FORM

Patient Name ____

Date Complaint Received ___________________________________

Account Number _______________________   Balance ___________________

Complaint ____

____

Action Taken To Resolve Complaint ___________________________

____

Manager Signature _______________________________   Date __________

Managers must concentrate on fostering human relations. They should create goodwill throughout the staff and incorporate good patient relations into collection procedures. The effects will go beyond the good graces of administration. It has been proven that the public responds much better to positive public relations, or goodwill collection techniques, than to a negative approach.

Answering Letters of Complaint

There is no magic formula for answering a complaint. Soothing the nerves and tempers of people who feel they have been inconvenienced, bothered, annoyed, or have lost time or money, and who have written to complain about their problems in no uncertain terms, takes considerable experience. There are persons who, by their very nature, are inclined to go out of their way to find something to complain about. These people should be treated kindly, sympathetically, and with respect.

They should be reassured by the form of expression of the person responding to the complaint that the medical group simply wishes to review the facts of the case, and that no one is trying to put anything over on them.

These practical pointers may prove valuable in answering a letter of complaint:

- Know the facts of the complaint. Carefully read the letter to find out precisely what it is the person is complaining about, why the person is complaining, and what he or she wants to be done to resolve the situation.

- Begin the letter of reply by thanking the person for taking the time to write to relate what is on his or her mind. After all, no office staff is perfect. Everybody involved can learn something of benefit if they are willing to listen with an open mind to the ideas or complaints of another person. Express appreciation for hearing from the patient.

- Whether patients who are complaining are right or wrong, tell them you are sorry and understand how they must feel.

- Explain what happened. If the person complaining is right and has a real reason to complain, explain what happened to cause the difficulty, what is being done or has been done to correct it, and what steps are being taken to make sure that the same thing will not happen again.

- Don't be too hard on the writer. If it turns out the person complaining is responsible for the problem, point this out, but do so tactfully.

- Don't downgrade or belittle patients who complain. Nothing is accomplished by riling them. After all, the goal is to keep peace.

- Don't try to be humorous. In answering a complaint, a lighthearted approach is the wrong approach entirely. A person who is dissatisfied about something, and who wants to convey this dissatisfaction, is in no mood for wit and humor.

- The answer to a complaint should be rather lengthy. A partial reply to a letter of complaint will not suffice. It may make the person feel that the problem is being sidestepped, which is reason enough to complain. A longer, more detailed response shows that the complaint is not being taken lightly.

- Beware of sounding sarcastic. In answering a letter of complaint, sarcasm is never appropriate. If, however, a letter of reply is not straightforward and down-to-earth, and if the letter does not have the proper tone, the reader may receive the impression that the writer is trying to be sarcastic.

- In closing a letter to the person complaining, be cordial and sincere. Ask for a final response to make sure the matter is closed. Tell them you want to be on friendly terms. After all, that is the whole reason for answering the complaint. Do not be surprised if the debtor responds to the letter in a very friendly and understanding manner.

- When people complaining are treated with respect, goodwill, and sincere appreciation, they often become the very best customers. Remember to try to make friends out of those who complain. Aim to see the situation from their point of view. Write the sort of letter you would like to receive if you were voicing a complaint and having a problem.

- Refer medical complaints to the physician who treated the patient or to the group's medical director.

Good Service Makes Dollars and Sense

Health care debtors, like all other debtors, search for reasons to avoid paying their bills. The medical group practice should not provide them with further excuses because of poor patient relations and improperly informed personnel. Unprofessional patient communication, such as poor customer service or unresolved complaints, is the fastest way to slow cash flow and turn away repeat business. Studies show that only 4 percent of dissatisfied customers will complain; 96 percent just walk away; and 91 percent will not return for repeat service.

An indifferent employee attitude is the most common form of unprofessional patient communication. Other employee "offenses" include: poorly informed employees, employees who are on the telephone while waiting on patients, employees who say an area of concern is not "my department," and employees who talk down to patients. These types of behavior can drive patients right out the door — some never to return. More importantly, once out the door, the average dissatisfied patient relates his or her dissatisfaction to over eight people. One in five dissatisfied patients will tell over 20 people! Poor customer service not only hurts the patient's view of the medical group, it can affect the opinions of others, too.

Another survey has found that it takes 12 positive actions to make up for one negative experience. However, seven out of ten patients will do future business with an organization if a grievance is fixed in their favor. When a complaint is resolved on the spot, 95 percent of patients will return. The faster a complaint is resolved, the faster a bill will be paid. Therefore, it is well worth the extra effort to make sure patient communication is always professional.

Skepticism is sometimes expressed that good collections and good patient relations can be accomplished simultaneously. However, it has been proven that patients respond best to good human relations. In other words, collections will improve when emphasis is placed on favorable patient relations throughout the collection system. Collections without favorable public relations will lead to complaints and will collect fewer dollars in the long run. Building a collection system that is consistent with good public relations is critical to the success of a collection program. Common public relations problems and recommended solutions are provided in *Figure 10-3*.

FIGURE 10-3.
PUBLIC RELATIONS PROBLEMS AND SOLUTIONS

COMMON PROBLEMS	**RECOMMENDED SOLUTIONS**
1. Poor quality of information from all points of patient registration.	• Put registration areas under control of the accounts receivable manager. • Monitor information and give feedback on errors, omissions, etc. Insist on quality at all points of registration. • Stress the importance of getting more information at registration. • Train the registration staff in collection, especially why information is required. • Verify critical information with copies of all identification or insurance cards. • Develop a good, productive preregistration program. • Use past information on patients — look it up.
2. Poor quality of bills and collection notices.	• Proofread bills and notices before mailing. • Review and rewrite all collection messages and notices. • Make all bills easy to read and understandable by the public. • Reduce late charges.
3. Lack of knowledge of what is done in the business office by internal departments.	• Have meetings with various departments to explain objectives in more detail. • Include a regular feature in an organization newsletter. • Hold an open house in the business office. • Communicate more regularly with administration and other department heads. • Invite them to staff meetings. • Make presentations at their meetings.
4. Lack of knowledge by the public of what to expect from the medical group.	• Place positive advertising in local newspapers and magazines, and have open houses. • Conduct educational classes for the public. • Give written handout material at registration. • Do a public relations survey by phone after service is rendered to go over charges, bills, collection policy, etc.
5. Poor service by business office staff.	• Train staff in technical areas and human relations. • Upgrade job requirements. • Update salaries and hire better people. • Give the staff incentives and recognition for good performance in public relations. • Reduce stress in the office and at registration points. • Have managers give more support to staff when public relations problems come up with administration.
6. Collection agency or outside attorney collection activity.	• Choose only the best after careful evaluation. • Monitor and audit on a regular basis. • Review collection notices and letters once a year.

The Fair Debt Collection Practices Act

The Fair Debt Collection Practices Act, which became law on March 20, 1978, was not designed to govern most medical collection activities. However, anyone who collects a debt in the same manner as a collection agency is subject to the requirements of this law.

If mailings are used to verify a debtor's location, any language or symbol indicating that the communication relates to the collection of a debt should be omitted from the stationery and envelope. Using a postcard to correct location information is also prohibited by the law. In locating a debtor, the collector is prohibited by law from communicating with a third party more than once, unless expressly requested to do so by that party, or the collector believes the first response was erroneous or incomplete.

Once the collector knows the consumer is represented by an attorney with respect to the debt and knows the name and address of that attorney, the collector must not communicate with anyone else, "unless the attorney fails to respond within a reasonable period of time." The law does not provide specific parameters for a "reasonable period of time." For protection of a medical group in lawsuits, it is good to establish a written office policy which can be used as a defense.

Within five days after the initial communication, the collector is obligated to send the debtor written verification of the amount of the debt, and the creditor to whom the debt is owed. If the debtor makes a written request for information or disputes any portion of the debt within 30 days, the collector must cease collection of the debt, or any disputed portion thereof. The Fair Credit Billing Act, part of the Consumer Credit Protection Act of 1968, defines guidelines similar to those specified in this section of the Fair Debt Collection Practices Act (American Collector's Association, Inc. 1979).

The law places limitations on communication with the debtor. Generally, the debt collector may only contact a patient between 8 A.M. and 9 P.M. in the debtor's time zone, unless the collector is aware that the patient works at night and sleeps during the day, or is otherwise inconvenienced by receiving communications during that time period. Collectors may not call patients at work if they know or have reason to know the debtor's employer prohibits such communications.

Once a consumer notifies the collector in writing that he or she refuses to pay the debt and wants communications stopped, the collector cannot pursue further communications except to advise the consumer that efforts are being terminated or to notify him or her that legal remedies may or will be invoked.

"A debt collector may not engage in any conduct for which the natural consequence is to harass, oppress, or abuse any person in connection with the collection of a debt," says the law (Ibid.). Six specific instances of abuse are expressly prohibited, but they are not all-inclusive. These are:

1. Use or threat of violence or other criminal means to harm the physical person, reputation, or property.

2.   Use of obscene, profane, or abusive language.

3.   Publication of "debtor lists." (Names of consumers who do not pay can be distributed to consumer reporting agencies.)

4.   Advertisement of the sale of any debt to coerce payment of the debt.

5.   Causing a telephone to ring or engaging any person in telephone conversation repeatedly or continuously with intent to annoy, abuse, or harass.

6.   Placement of telephone calls without meaningful disclosure of the caller's identity.

The law prohibits any false representation intended to mislead the debtor, such as distorting company documents in such a way as to make the reader believe they are legal documents, falsifying the collector's identity, misstating the nature or status of a debt, or any other misleading designations.

Some unfair practices are specifically prohibited by the law, including such practices as depositing a postdated check prior to the date on the check; causing collect charges on a telephone bill, telegram expenses, or other costs to be made to the consumer; or using a post card to communicate with a consumer.

The Fair Debt Collection Practices Act is enforced both administratively and judicially. The Federal Trade Commission can treat a violation of the act as an unfair or deceptive practice under the law. Violators are also subject to civil penalties in federal and state courts.

**SUMMARY OF
KEY STRATEGY 10**

When developing a total collection program in a medical group, these points merit consideration:

1. Favorable public relations are critical to any successful collection program and are good both for a medical group's public image and for recovery of dollars.

2. Good public relations do not just happen. It takes a serious effort to incorporate an overall strategy into a medical group and to train personnel to follow guidelines.

3. A training program and frequent refreshers are good morale boosters for staff and will pay rich dividends.

4. Favorable or unfavorable public relations in a health care collection program are also determined by policies, procedures, practices, notices, and letters.

5. A collection policy should be developed taking into account medical group philosophy, and steps should be taken to make sure **everyone** is aware of it — staff and public.

6. Collection procedures that complement policy should be developed by asking, "What effect will this procedure have on public relations?"

7. Cracks not covered by policy and procedures can be filled by making sure staff uses appropriate collection practices to avoid poor public relations.

8. The wording, design, and image of collection notices and letters should prompt attention and evoke a positive reaction, not create hostility or confusion that will lead to public relations problems.

KEY STRATEGY 11:
SET GOALS FOR DIRECTION, MOTIVATION, AND RESULTS

The involvement of staff members in goal setting and the implementation of some simple, proven job enrichment techniques can help to improve cash flow in a medical group. Both approaches encourage development of teamwork attitudes, improve staff morale, and increase motivation. Best of all, with proper leadership by the administrator, staff will produce results to lower outstanding revenue.

Goal Setting

One of the key ingredients to successful collections is goal setting. Whether an individual is responsible for personal performance and results, or is in a supervisory role eliciting results from others, goal setting can bring amazing success.

Arthur S. Hummel, an attorney, licensed insurance executive, vice president in the brokerage firm of Mosely, Hallgarten & Estabrook, Inc., and director of Mosely Financial Counseling Services, is a believer in setting goals. "Too many guys — top guys — talk in generalities [about getting organized]," Hummel explains. "Tomorrow. Always tomorrow. But they never get around to getting their goals in order. And all the while, factors beyond their control are pecking away at them." Hummel urges us to establish goals and then determine how they can be accomplished.

Bud Selig, successful president of the Milwaukee Brewers, defines his own personal limits by setting goals and reaching for success:

> I want happiness and success. Maybe not for the same reasons that other people do. I want success for a job well done. This experience I've had in baseball, almost 15 years now, six years trying to get a team under very diverse circumstances, was frustrating because I was turned down several times.
>
> I'll never forget the night we got the club, the feeling I had inside of me. It is hard to describe. I really did feel fulfilled, not only for myself, but for everyone else that worked so hard, too. It showed me a lot about life — tenacity, the ability to set your goal on something even if it seems very high.
>
> It's said that there has to be a place in the world for the mediocre. Well, sure, but everybody has some ability, in some area, in some way, and I really believe those who have the drive, the inner strength to motivate themselves and continue to motivate themselves, will experience the fullness of life.

It's very easy to get discouraged. You have to be able to recognize what your strengths are and what your limitations are and then do the best you can within those boundaries.

Think Success

To be successful, a person must think success. The staff of a credit department must have a common goal for which they all are striving. They must take pride in the excellence of their work. A person's attitude toward the job not only governs individual progress, but also affects the attitudes and progress of every fellow worker and, in turn, affects the entire department.

However, managers cannot motivate their workers. The manager's job is to ensure that working conditions enable workers to motivate themselves. Although this may sound confusing, it becomes clearer upon consideration that a manager's job is to create an environment that allows people to become motivated. Managers create the mood, environment, and opportunities within their departments or organizations to allow motivation to occur within individuals.

An entire chapter of *In Search of Excellence*, by Thomas J. Peters and Robert H. Waterman, Jr., is devoted to motivation: "Productivity through People." Some of the major points covered in that chapter may be appropriate to the medical group manager who is attempting to develop a motivational climate within his or her own organization (Peters and Waterman, 1982, p. 235-278).

- **"People will flood you with ideas if you let them."** Peters and Waterman point out that people have many ideas and are willing to express them if we simply ask for their input. This can be done in staff meetings, one-on-one discussions, special assignments, and by creating an atmosphere that encourages people to come forth with their ideas.

- **"Treat people as partners and with respect."** The authors are not referring to becoming "buddies" with employees, but instead, treating them as partners in the business. This includes almost every aspect of management, which reflects the notion that employees should be viewed as partners in every enterprise. They should be treated with the same respect that would be given to a full partner.

- **"Celebrate achievement through corny, unabashed hoopla."** To obtain results, an atmosphere of excitement should be created, and results will be achieved. The authors point out that successful organizations add excitement to their work environments and are not afraid to stir up a little "hoopla."

- **"Make sure your people feel needed."** Peters and Waterman point out that successful companies make sure all feel they are needed. Each employee is essential to the overall success of the department and the organization as a whole. All contributions are appreciated; each is an integral part of the organization's success. It is the manager's job to make sure each employee realizes that his or her efforts and accomplishments are needed.

- **"Provide incentives."** Successful organizations, the authors point out, provide incentives — not necessarily financial rewards. Incentives come in a number of different shapes and sizes. Three important factors must be kept in mind: (1) performance incentives should be worthwhile; (2) managers should facilitate employees' efforts to attain those goals; and (3) rewards should be publicized both before and after they have been won.

- **"Celebrate victories."** Successful organizations make a point of celebrating when they win. When a victory has been accomplished in any aspect of receivables management, the accomplishment should be celebrated. Office get-togethers for coffee and rolls, wine and cheese parties, and celebrations away from the office (such as dinners, picnics, cookouts, and things of that nature) should be regular occurrences. The main point is — celebrate!

- **"Commitment to quality."** Interestingly enough, emphasis on quality will also improve productivity. After all, increased quality saves time and effort down the road. Managers can actually improve staff morale and motivation by stressing the importance of quality in all aspects of each job. Emphasizing development of self-pride in every aspect of an employee's job will heighten quality awareness, improve productivity, and stimulate motivation.

These points, brought out not only in the chapter cited but in various sections throughout the book, illustrate the approaches of successful companies to motivation. The motivational tactics described here and elsewhere in Peters and Waterman's book can be creatively applied to any medical group setting.

Managing Change

The changing environment within health care accounts receivable challenges managers not only to manage change, but to manage people during change. A recent book focuses on companies that have proven successful at managing change and managing their people within a changing environment. In *The Change Masters*, Rosabeth Moss Kanter points out what innovative companies do to motivate their employees during a period of change (Kanter 1983, p. 129-155). The following are highlights from a chapter entitled "Cultures of Pride, Climates of Success: Incentives for Enterprise in High-Income Companies."

- **"Be open minded — willing to listen to and encourage ideas."** Here, the author stresses obtaining ideas from staff members, much like the authors of *In Search of Excellence*. People managing change in successful companies have a clear idea of what they are being asked to do. Managers can and should make sure their staff members have a clear understanding of what is expected of them in terms of objectives, goals, and assignments. Successful managers prompt input from staff members to help them solve problems.

- **"Encourage reaching — provide action incentives."** A reminder is in order: by developing incentives — incentives that mean something to the performers — we encourage self-pride in workers and create a motivational climate. These incentives need not be after the fact. Providing an opportunity to launch an idea into action is often incentive enough for workers to make a project successful. It is, after all, their "baby."

- **"People feel they belong to a meaningful entity and can realize value by their contributions."** Self-pride perpetuates itself as workers see their contributions adding to the "big picture." Because the organization helped them succeed, workers want to make sure the organization prospers. Workers feel a sense of community pride; they are all working toward a common goal — success.

- **"Pride in the organization — establish innovation as mainstream rather than countercultural."** Organizations that are open to ideas create a sense of self-pride within workers and worker pride in the company. Because innovative organizations allow workers to voice their ideas and concerns, their people know that their input is not just expected, but essential to overall development and progress. Because their voices matter, workers are more willing to come forward with ideas and suggestions.

- **"Prompt open communication as air waves for innovation — encourage face-to-face communication up, down, and sideways."** Each part of an organization is dependent upon the success of the other parts. Therefore, open communication among sections, departments, and individuals is fundamental to success within each, as well as success of the whole.

- **"Energize the grass-roots employee — get him involved in planning and action of meaningful projects — participative management."** Expecting employees to be innovative without presenting them with a problem to solve is tantamount to asking someone to fix something that is not broken. Workers should be challenged to develop a new perspective, to question procedures. They will present the problem and together with management possible actions can be outlined, but it is important to let workers test their plans and present their final designs. When workers are allowed to implement innovations, they will learn and be enriched by the experience. The group will be a step ahead, and the management approach will have proven itself effective.

Though the points presented here are ideas for management within industrial firms, they may easily be adapted to the medical group practice situation. In fact, with the number of changes occurring within health care management, innovative ideas are essential to ensure survival. These items are mentioned only to encourage creativity in designing a unique motivational climate that is appropriate for a particular organization.

Motivation and Success

Individual and departmental goal setting is the key to motivating staff and improving performance. Goal setting is also the foundation of the points mentioned in *In Search of Excellence* and *The Change Masters*.

"People really don't want to work these days!" Hundreds of business owners, managers, and supervisors, especially those in smaller firms, are voicing this concern and searching for ways to motivate employees. Edward Pickett, who for

10 years worked in industry providing management training for employees of private firms before joining the University of Wisconsin as a professor, has developed a course focusing on motivation. Pickett, who later became the coordinator of statewide education extension network programs, has noted a five-year study and analysis of 150 new Wisconsin businesses showing that one of the major people problems of business is employee motivation. "The older theories of motivation aren't working anymore," contends Pickett. "Salary is not the motivator it used to be; yet some people are motivated by it. Motivation is within people — the manager's role is to provide the climate for its growth."

Employees are keenly interested in earning a positive performance appraisal. It is only natural. Positive evaluations may have some effect on pay, not only by bringing about merit increases, but also by advancing employees to new jobs that include increases of power and responsibility along with more money. Success, then, is a common goal for most employees.

Eugene Jennings is even more emphatic. He refers to the drive for success as the "success ethic" and says that it is self-fueling — that is, the more you get, the more you want. Motivation is goal-directed behavior. Setting meaningful goals and achieving them increases self-motivation, both for the individual and for the staff, and motivation is what makes the cash register ring for a group's collection efforts.

Managing by objectives, job enrichment, organizational development, and perhaps behavior modification are all different parts of the same cloth aimed at making organizations effective. Once it becomes clear that the span of control goes beyond one person, the professional manager will be on the road to success.

Management by Objectives

Management by objectives sets the scene for identifying the importance of goals and how they should be ordered. It is a directional approach dependent upon commitment. Objectives are set and management decisions are centered around them. Organizing, forecasting, planning, communication, and measuring staff effectiveness by results are all facets of this management tool.

The blueprint that follows is a simple, effective version of management by objectives with guidelines for individual or team goal setting that can be implemented by a medical group. This process will help in targeting areas that are critical to improvement of cash flow within a group. *Figure 11-1* provides an overview of the sequence of actions for management by objectives.

Pinpoint key result areas. Prior to listing the most important job components, the written job description should be reviewed in detail. Those words that describe, in a few words, specific areas of responsibility should be circled or underlined. If no written job description exists, responsibilities as they are understood should be described in writing. The tasks and activities that seem to occupy the bulk of time on a day-to-day basis should be noted as well.

FIGURE 11-1.
SEQUENCE OF ACTIONS FOR MANAGEMENT BY OBJECTIVES

SEQUENCE	ACTION
#1	Pinpoint key result areas (components of the job that are most important).
#2	Designate percentage levels of importance for the key result areas chosen in sequence #1.
#3	Develop performance indicators for each key result area (measurements of performance in each area).
#4	Set specific short-range and long-range goals for the indicators.
#5	Develop an action plan.

It is impossible to evaluate an administrator or employee without knowing the results he or she is expected to effect in key areas. With the above information as a base, a simple listing can be made of major areas of responsibility and key result areas using the following guidelines:

* Use one to four words to describe each area, such as cash flow, staff development, bad debt, budget, collections, self-development, quality control, purchasing, record keeping, agency placements, profits, billings, expenses, public relations, registrations, job enrichment, among others.

* Avoid stating quantities or time allotments such as "increase," "maximize," or "satisfy" in key result areas.

Additionally, each completed listing of eight or less key result areas should:

* Be directly associated with overall objectives
* Indicate the core responsibilities of the position
* Be within the active limits of the job description
* Represent a total of 100 percent of the output, not input, of the position
* Avoid unnecessary overlap with other job positions

No listing should be so superficial that job responsibilities are not defined and that goals are not set, or so detailed and cumbersome that the planning process is inhibited and the job description set down is unreasonable. Collectively, the listings should include all responsibilities necessary to obtain the end result. The next step is to assign the percentage level of importance to each area. A form for pinpointing key result areas is provided in *Worksheet 8* in Appendix A.

Designate percentage levels of importance. The next step is to assign a percentage level to each key result area in terms of its importance to the total area of responsibility. The cumulative figure should equal 100 percent.

Establish performance indicators. To establish effective performance indicators for any job responsibility, this question must be answered in specific terms: What indicators tell administrators a good job is being done? The following guidelines may be helpful in determining the best answer to this question.

Performance indicators should be defined:

- For each separate job responsibility

- In seven words or less

- In neutral, descriptive terms that are easily measured

- In specific terms (ambiguous or vague language may mislead or be misinterpreted by the reader)

- Without using "and," "or," "etc.," commas, semicolons, colons, dashes, slashes, or other connectives

Some examples of performance indicators for the medical group accounts receivable manager are:

- Monthly outstanding bookings
- Percentage of bad debt to gross charges
- Percentage of bad debt to net charges
- Number of complaints voiced to administration
- Gross collection ratio
- Percentage variance of actual expenses to budget
- Average monthly collections
- Average time span from charge to billing
- Total outstanding dollars
- Number of billings per week
- Dollars billed per week or per month
- Dollars outstanding as a percentage of accounts receivable
- Gross collection ratio by financial class
- Net collection ratio by financial class

Set goals. Because an organization exists for a purpose — to provide a service or to produce a product — goals are a part of any working situation. Goals encourage us to reach our potential and go beyond.

The essential features of a sound goal are that it must be specific, measurable, significant, and achievable within the defined time span at a certain cost. An examination of key result areas will help in determining the necessary levels of performance and types of duties they suggest. This information is essential to formulating short-range and long range goals. Results should be reviewed, and suggestions for improvement should be centered around the findings. Short-term goals can be adjusted as necessary to achieve the desired long-term results.

These six questions should be asked to determine whether each established goal is sound:

1. Is it measurable in tangible terms such as collection totals, outstanding accounts receivable, or percentage of bad debt?

2. Under what terms is it measurable — as a percentage, actual, net, gross, or other?

3. Is it result centered? Does the goal require achievement of a specific end?

4. Taking the medical group's needs and available resources into account, is it realistic and attainable?

5. Is it time related? Practical deadlines are important when one works toward a specific goal (for instance, a reduction in accounts receivable of $100,000 by June 30, monthly bookings of three months by June 30, or bad debt write-off down to two percent by June 30).

6. Is it within the individual or staff's competence and experience, or is additional training needed?

Develop an action plan. The final step of the management by objectives process is to use the short-range and long-range goals as a foundation for development of an action plan. The action plan serves as a "road map" for accomplishing goals.

Figure 11-2, *Figure 11-3*, and *Figure 11-4* are designed to continue the sequence of actions outlined in *Figure 11-1*. *Worksheet 9*, in Appendix A, provides a form for determining key result areas and performance indicators. *Worksheet 10* provides a monthly goal status report form, and *Worksheet 11* provides an annual action plan form.

FIGURE 11-2.
SAMPLE KEY RESULT AREAS AND PERFORMANCE INDICATORS

PREPARED BY <u>Group Administrator</u>   DATE <u>1/1/X1</u>

Key Result Area / Level of Importance	Performance Indicator	Acceptable Result	Expected Result	Possible Result
Accounts Receivable (50%)*	Months self-pay outstanding	3.7 months (by 12/30/X1)	3.5 months (by 12/30/X1)	3 months (by 12/30/X1)
	Medicare and Medicaid outstanding	$25,000 over 120 days (by 12/30/X1)	$15,000 over 120 days (by 12/30/X1)	$5,000 over 120 days (by 12/30/X1)
	Gross collection ratio	90%	92%	95%
Quality Control (10%)*	Percent of action plan completed (audits and procedure review)	75%	80%	90%
Staff Development (10%)*	Percent of action plan completed	75%	80%	90%
Bad Debt (10%)*	Percent of write-off of gross revenue	4.5% year-to-date	4% year-to-date	3.5% year-to-date
Expense Control (5%)*	Variance of actual expenses to budget	0.5% over budget (by 12/30/X1)	On budget (by 12/30/X1)	2% under budget (by 12/30/X1)
Public Relations (15%)*	Complaints to administration	2	1	0

*Percentage level of importance

FIGURE 11-3.
SAMPLE COMPLETED MONTHLY GOAL STATUS REPORT

PREPARED BY <u>Group Administrator</u>   DATE <u>1/1/X1</u>   PERIOD <u>11/1/X0 to 11/30/X0</u>

Key Result Area Level of Importance	Performance Indicator	Acceptable Result	Expected Result	Possible Result	Status at Month End
Accounts Receivable (50%)*	Actual self-pay monthly outstanding bookings	3.7 months	3.5 months	3.0 months	3.65 months
Quality control (10%)*	Percent of action plan completed (audits and procedure review year-to-date)	75%	80%	90%	75%
Staff development (10%)*	Percent of action plan completed year-to-date	75%	80%	90%	90%
Bad debt (10%)*	Percent of write-off to revenue year-to-date	5%	4.5%	4%	4.5%
Expense control (5%)*	Variance of actual expenses to budget year-to-date	0.5% over budget	On budget	0.5% under budget	0.5% over budget
Public relations (15%)*	Complaints to administration per month year-to-date	2	1	0	1

*Percentage level of importance

FIGURE 11-4.
SAMPLE COMPLETED ANNUAL ACTION PLAN

Prepared by <u>Group Administrator</u>   Date <u>12/31/X1</u>   Period <u>1/1/X1 to 12/31/X1</u>

Key Result Area	Goal	Projections — Action Planned	Projections — Commencing date-Completion Date	Actual — Date Action Taken	Actual — Comments: Including Reasons for Action Not Taken or Changes in Plan
Accounts Receivable	Reduce self-pay outstanding to 3 months of billings	Review monthly aged trial balance (ATB) and monitor accounts (complete by midmonth)	Begin 1/X1	01/15/X1 02/17/X1 03/15/X1 04/18/X1 05/15/X1 06/17/X1 07/16/X1 08/14/X1 09/15/X1 10/16/X1 11/18/X1 12/14/X1	Implemented
		Review aged trial balance, pull accounts and work accounts exceeding $500	7/15/X1	07/15/X1 08/14/X1 09/15/X1 10/16/X1 11/18/X1 12/14/X1	Implemented
		Daily, review any applications for credit to determine arrangements	7/15/X1	07/15/X1 and daily thereafter	Implemented
		Monitor strict adherence to billing schedule	7/15/X1	07/2/X1	Implemented 2 weeks early
		Initiate and maintain maternity deposits	4/15/X1	04/15/X1	Implemented
		Review billing report daily	1/1/X1	01/1/X1	Implemented
		Initiate and review daily report of insurance accounts not verified	8/1/X1	07/25/X1	Implemented 1 week early
		Complete review of credit card payments and procedures	5/1/X1	06/3/X1	Review delayed one month, business office personnel required additional training
		Install cash drawer in registration area	1/15/X1	08/30/X1	Delayed because of complications

Setting Goals with Staff

Discussion of goal setting leads naturally to the art of managing patient accounts. Development of goals with staff can be helpful in motivating, directing, and controlling the accounts receivable staff toward success in improving a medical group's cash flow, even during poor economic conditions. In short, it is one of the best ways to ensure results.

Almost any point of attack to improve collections may be included in staff goal-setting meetings. Goals may be developed regarding monthly collection totals in outstanding accounts receivable for any given time in the future, number or dollar amount billed in a week or month, or amount collected by cashiers during a certain time frame.

Developing goals for outstanding accounts receivable and collections can be a real challenge. However, goals give direction to the entire staff, make work considerably more interesting and rewarding for everyone, and allow staff efforts to become more profitable for the medical group as a whole.

After members of the administrative staff have determined goals and set collection standards, the entire staff may be invited to contribute ideas for lowering receivables and reaching overall goals. Brainstorming sessions are great for generating ideas. Staff participation in goal setting leads to substantial improvements in performance. The impact of a well-developed goal-setting program in a department should become apparent within a few months.

Reports generated from the goal-setting process will provide tight control and a substantiated overall picture. These reports also provide staff with feedback and a sense of achievement, recognition, and accomplishment.

The following are hypothetical situations in which a medical group is determining goals and standards for certain collection categories.

Case Study 1. Let us assume you were to develop goals for the total outstanding balance in each major financial category within your receivables. This is the formula you might choose:

> **Third Party**
> Present Outstanding: $330,000
> Goal: $224,000
> Amount to Reduce: $106,000

If you billed an average of $60,000 a week over the past two months, the present outstanding balance would reflect five and one-half weeks' average outstanding billings in third party. The goal of $224,000 would reflect about four weeks' billings. If you are to gain ground and reach your goal, you naturally must collect more than you bill over the next several months. So, a projected guideline is set:

Comparison of Third-Party Billings to Collection Goal
Average Billings per Week: $60,000
Average Collection Goal per Week: $65,000
Gain in One Month: $20,000

CONCLUSION: Adjust collection goals to $65,000 a week to reach the projection of reducing third-party accounts receivable by $106,000 in a little over five months.

Medicaid
Present Outstanding: $235,000
Goal: $154,000
Amount to Reduce: $ 81,000

You averaged $15,000 a week over the last two months in Medicaid billings, with a monthly average of $60,000. Due to the normal delay in payment, if you bill $60,000 in January, it will be paid in March. This means you usually carry a minimum of two full months of billings ($60,000 + $60,000 = $120,000). Additionally, you get rejections each month that tie up billings. You can expect that Medicaid will reject payment on claims in the amount of another $5,000 to $15,000 each month. So, you can expect an additional amount of receivables in Medicaid to average about $10,000 each month.

Therefore, the minimum you can expect to carry in Medicaid is $140,000 ($60,000 + $60,000 + $20,000), plus 10 percent for fluctuation, bringing the total to $154,000 ($140,000 + $14,000).

Self-Pay
Present Outstanding: $148,000
Goal: $100,000
Amount to Reduce: $ 48,000

Over the last two months you averaged $15,000 in billings for self-pay accounts per week, including insurance rejections. The present outstanding balance reflects approximately ten weeks of billings. The goal of $100,000 would reflect about six weeks' worth of outstanding patient liability collections. Your goals could be set up as such.

Comparison of Current Self-Pay Billings to Collection Goal
Average Billings per Week: $15,000
Average Collection Goal per Week: $20,000
Gain in One Month: $20,000

CONCLUSION: Adjust collection standard in patient liability to $20,000 a week in collections until receivables are lowered and reach a total of $100,000. Then you can readjust collection standards to equal billings if you want patient liability collections to stay at that $100,000 figure.

Determining your goal for outstanding bookings from this formula might be based on another hypothetical case.

Case Study 2. First, determine average weekly billings over the past two months in each category:

AVERAGE WEEKLY BILLINGS

COLLECTION CATEGORY	AMOUNT
Self-pay	$20,000
Third party	$65,000
Medicare	$60,000
Medicaid	$20,000
Blue Cross/Blue Shield	$60,000
Other	$34,000

Then, determine a reasonable turnaround time for each category. For instance, suppose Blue Cross/Blue Shield reimbursements should be turning around in three weeks from the date of billing. The goal for carrying Blue Cross/Blue Shield billings would be three weeks (3 X $60,000 = $180,000). Here is a summary of category goals:

STANDARD FOR ACCOUNTS RECEIVABLE CATEGORIES

COLLECTION CATEGORY	TIME CARRIED/AMOUNT PER WEEK	TOTAL
Self-pay	10 weeks x $20,000	$200,000
Third party	5 weeks x $65,000	$325,000
Medicare	3 weeks x $60,000	$180,000
Medicaid	8 weeks x $20,000	$160,000
Blue Cross/Blue Shield	3 weeks x $60,000	$180,000
Other	3 weeks x $34,000	$102,000

TOTAL ACCOUNTS RECEIVABLE GOAL $1,147,000[*]

[*]HMO receivables should be cleared out of the aged trial balance as soon as possible and are not shown in this example.

After goals have been determined and collection standards set, the entire staff may be invited to come up with ideas for decreasing receivables and reaching overall goals. For instance, a specific collection strategy might be developed with staff input, after zeroing in on each category of outstanding collectibles and drawing ideas from staff. A sample is provided in *Figure 11-5*.

Developing standards in accounts receivable can motivate staff and add excitement to everyone's job — and bring a medical group one step closer to achieving collection goals. These points outline the essence of goal setting:

* Specific, challenging goals lead to better performance.

* Feedback on goal-directed activities motivates staff to heighten performance.

FIGURE 11-5.
SAMPLE COLLECTION STRATEGY

Collection Category	Ideas to Decrease Accounts Receivable
Self-pay	• Tighten control at time of service. • Restrict courtesy write-offs. • Keep financial arrangements firm and follow up with patients. • Improve preregistration control; have up-to-date preregistration; verify commercial insurance and financial arrangements when necessary. • Accept credit card payments at time of service.
Third party	• Verify insurance coverage during patient registration. • Encourage patients to pay at time of service and to file their own claims with their insurers. • Tighten follow-up to 45 days where feasible on larger balances.
Medicare	• Follow up unapproved Medicare to move accounts into billing stage. • Hold down errors in billing and returned billings — improve quality control. • Tighten billing on approved accounts to 14 days, or under if account balance exceeds $200. • Copy Medicare card for each billing.
Medicaid	• Follow up after monthly remittance. • Increase employee and patient understanding of the program through employee education. • Allow fewer errors in billing.

- Comparative feedback (actual to goal) provides the worker with a sense of achievement, recognition, and accomplishment.

- Goals set jointly by employee and supervisor lead to substantial improvement in performance.

- Healthy competition increases productivity.

- Setting specific goals significantly increases productivity.

The following worksheets are presented in Appendix A for application of analytical methods to actual accounts receivable: *Worksheet 12 — Comparative Analysis of Actual to Projected Goal, Worksheet 13 — Formula to Reach Goal, Worksheet 14 — Collector's Monthly Status Report*, and *Worksheet 15 — Accounts Receivable Status Report*.

Job Enrichment in Practice

The final component in this strategy for improved collections is job enrichment. The principle of job enrichment refers to the process of analyzing job content to determine if jobs can be arranged so that individuals have more interesting and challenging tasks; greater responsibilities; more opportunities for growth, development, and advancements; and greater recognition for achievements. By constructing and implementing work modules, practicing vertical loading, and developing feedback mechanisms, medical groups not only improve the quality of the working situation of their employees, but may also be increasing daily and long-range overall productivity.

One of the most useful approaches in job enrichment is to look for natural, whole units of work, or work modules. A close look at the overall work flow system may help in determining what natural units of work might coexist within separate departments. Some areas that may lend themselves to this concept are the billing, collection, and registration areas. Billers could bill all third-party payers as well as patients by splitting up the alphabet among them. The same idea would apply to collectors and their follow-ups with insurance companies and patients.

Another concept pertinent to discussion of work modules is the team approach to collections. Linking compatible workers in the reception area, collection department, and billing department to form joint goals and deal with the same section of the group's patient load will serve several purposes. First, each team will learn the specifics of certain patient accounts. Second, members of each team will encourage one another as they work toward their joint goals. Third, contacts concerning specific patient accounts will be directed only to one of those team members, incorporating good public relations for the group and making workloads manageable for employees.

Vertical loading is another form of job enrichment. In this approach, planning, decision making, and problem solving are transferred as far down the organizational ladder as possible. More responsibilities are passed on to cashiers, billers, collectors, and registration staff to encourage production. Group leaders can be appointed to act as liaisons in relaying questions or problems to supervisors.

Patient representatives may also play a role in the success of collectors, billers, and registration personnel in meeting collection goals. Since patient representatives are knowledgeable about the personal needs of each patient, they may know the best way to approach a patient concerning a bill. However, they should not be directly involved in the contact, since that is not their primary function. Feedback from the patient through the representative may also be beneficial to overall goal planning and policy design.

Feedback mechanisms are a third area of job enrichment. Because we frequently find people unable to determine for themselves how well they are doing their jobs, feedback on results of staff efforts is an essential ingredient to developing employee motivation. Time should be taken to search for ways to convey directly to staff the results of their efforts. This might take the form of reports showing figures such as billing totals by biller, collection totals by cashier, collection totals by collector, or outstanding accounts receivable by collector. These reports can be routed through memos, posted, or brought out at staff meetings. The bottom line is: Give special recognition where it is deserved!

Job enrichment can increase staff morale, lead to improved self-motivation, and, in the end, bring home the desired results — reduction of outstanding bookings. *Figure 11-6* provides a recap of approaches to job enrichment.

FIGURE 11-6.
APPROACHES TO JOB ENRICHMENT

Work Modules (natural, whole units of work)	• Billers — by alphabetical break-out • Collectors — by alphabetical break-out • Team concept — collector/cashier/biller
Vertical Loading (more decision making is transferred down the line)	• Billers • Collectors • Patient representatives • Group leaders
Feedback Mechanisms	• Goal status reports by individuals • Reports by individuals • Billing reports by billers • Outstanding balance reports by collectors

SUMMARY OF KEY STRATEGY 11	To add enthusiasm and direction to a medical group collection program, a goal-setting process should be developed that:

1. Will allow setting of meaningful goals in the right areas to increase collections and maintain favorable public relations with the most cost-effective methods.

2. Gets the entire staff involved and committed.

3. Provides feedback to everyone involved.

4. Is closely monitored, tracked, and reported, and allows for recognition of achievements.

5. Provides the most rewarding form of employee motivation.

KEY STRATEGY 12:
MAXIMIZE COLLECTION AGENCY RECOVERY

The use of collection agencies is an important link in the chain of a strong collection program, depending on the size of the collection staff. The smaller the staff, the more the medical group depends on them to play an active role in increasing total cash flow.

Traditionally, medical group practices go outside to professional collectors. Recently, however, there has been a move toward in-house setups. This key strategy will explain how to get the most out of external collection agencies, and the advantages, disadvantages, and setup of an internal collection agency. The choice of an agency and how well it performs can make a considerable difference in overall collection results and patient relations of a medical group.

Use of Outside Agencies

An accounts receivable manager would not think of releasing an account to an outside agency before proper effort has been made to collect it within the medical group's system. By the same token, at a certain point it becomes fruitless to continue to spend time and money trying to collect overdue accounts within the accounts receivable department. Usually, when pursuit is no longer profitable to the medical group, managers choose to submit the account to an outside collection firm.

There are several major points to consider when analyzing accounts receivable before referring them to an agency for collection. These are:

1. The economies of submitting the bill to an outside firm.
2. The time lapse involved.
3. The public relations problems an outside collection agency can create.

Economic factors. Two important economic questions should be asked before submitting any account to a collection agency:

1. Are the agency's fees reasonable when contrasted with internal collection costs?
2. Is the probability of collecting greater with an agency than it is with the internal accounts receivable staff?

This formula is not new. However, the more accurately a manager determines the costs of internal collection and estimates the probability of staff collecting the account, the closer he or she will come to determining the most effective time to discontinue internal collection efforts and turn the account over to an agency.

Many medical group administrators or patient accounts managers find themselves constantly fighting an uphill battle with overdue receivables. They never stop mounting! There is no turnoff for extending medical credit. Decisiveness is crucial when turning accounts over to a collection agency. The costs of collecting accounts make a difference in net recovery rates. From an economic viewpoint, when internal collection costs make net recovery less than what is expected from an agency, it is time to refer the account to outside professional collectors.

Time factors. Since most medical group administrators are limited in the amount of time they or their staff can spend on accounts, there should be a fixed policy for referring aged accounts after a certain period. Firm decisions must be made. In some cases, this might be 120 days after service, the month after service, or six to eight months after service is rendered. In any case, an account should never age a year before being turned over to an agency unless there are unusual factors involved.

An extended time lapse may make an account uncollectible. When an account is allowed to age without proper follow-up, it usually becomes much more difficult to collect, by staff or anyone, and this is particularly true in the area of medical collections. Statistics show the greater the gap between medical service and payment, the less likely an account will be collected in full, if at all. Patients may move, become unemployed, become ill again, take on excessive obligations, or may decide they were dissatisfied with the service or physician. The key is to keep collection efforts consistent and timely.

Public relations factors. Of course, in dealing with medical accounts, economic and time factors are certainly not the only considerations to weigh in referring accounts for third-party collection. There is the important aspect of patient relations. This is a critical consideration for any medical group office today. Strange as it sounds, if difficult and troublesome accounts with poor paying habits are to be collected with success and good public relations are to be maintained, proper handling of the account by some outside or third party is necessary.

Proper handling, however polite and courteous, often arouses a patient's anger. This anger will usually be pointed toward the one who did the telephoning or corresponding. Involvement of a collection agency, that perhaps has personnel better equipped to handle these type of accounts, can help protect the image of a medical group. If some of the indignation does come back to the group on an account that is with a third party, the group's image can actually be improved by explaining the position and thus gaining favor in the patient's eyes.

Occasionally, and probably more often in medical accounts than commercial, there is the nagging temptation to write off an account and discontinue all collection efforts rather than refer to a third party for collection. It is important to think twice before doing so. This approach has drawbacks. For instance, word gets around of a medical group's unwillingness to take all possible steps to collect. If this is the group policy, it invariably becomes known to the chronic "debtors" who begin to come to the group more often than to other groups more persistent in collection. A reputation of this nature can increase collection costs considerably.

Secondly, this approach is not fair to paying patients. Why should they be asked to pay for today's increasing medical costs when the group does not make every effort to collect from others? From a realistic point of view, in the long run someone must pay for those who do not. An indirect result may be increased charges. With the alarming rise in medical costs, all factors in holding back cost must be considered.

Selection Criteria

The most important element to consider in choosing a third party to service accounts is the financial integrity of the organization. The best indicator of integrity is a long record of ethical dealings with other clients, particularly medical group practices and other health care providers.

There are several other factors to consider in selecting a third-party collector, including the following:

- Accurate accounting and reporting of all funds collected for the medical group
- Prompt remittance of those collections due
- Public or patient relations
- Good and willing service for special requests and reports
- Satisfactory net recovery rate
- Understanding of the special nature of medical accounts

Whatever third party is chosen for the service of delinquent accounts, it is important to remember that this organization will be handling the medical group's money. The third party can be held to be acting as the group's agent, and the group is responsible for its actions.

References should always be obtained from the agency under consideration. The names of other companies, medical institutions, and professional people whom the agency is servicing should be requested. Then, follow-up is essential.

The American Collectors Association makes the following observations in the selection of a collection agency:

1. The agency should show evidence of having complied with any state or local bonding or licensing provisions.

2. It should be a member of an international trade association, such as the American Collectors Association.

3. Reputation is a vital consideration. One of the most important ways to select an agency is by checking those for whom it personally collects.

4. A personal visit to the office may provide valuable information. The business setup and form letters should be noted.

It is important to determine if the agency segregates medical accounts from the other accounts. An agency should be able to separate medical accounts so that they can be handled in a different manner than accounts from a utility company, department store, or other retailer. Medical accounts should be handled by a specialist who is familiar with medical charges, terminology, health insurance, and health factors. Medical collections are different and should be collected with this difference in mind.

It is recommended that only one or two agencies be utilized. This simplifies accounting when applying the money and eases referral procedures. There is also less confusion about who has the account when a payment is received. It is best to use two collection agencies for referrals. They can be put in competition with each other, and the agency providing the best net recovery can be rewarded with two-thirds of the business.

Commissions and Recovery Rate

Agencies usually accept accounts for collection on a contingent fee basis. If there is no collection, there is no charge. They charge a commission only on funds actually collected. There is no charge on accounts which are listed and for which the agency does not obtain results.

Some agencies try to sell on an escalating contingency rate after placement. The older the account gets, the harder it is to collect, so the contingency rate increases as the account ages at the agency. This only provides an incentive to collect accounts slowly. However, some agencies will give reduced rates for early placements. The older the account is when placed, the higher the fee.

The agency should be notified promptly of any payments received by the medical group on accounts which have been placed with the agency, so the agency will not be attempting to collect an account previously paid. Failure to do so can result in costly public relations problems. Whether the accounts are paid to the medical group or paid to the agency, the agency expects its commission.

Contingent fee commissions charged by agencies will range from about 25 to 40 percent. Accounts previously handled by other agencies, accounts which require legal action, or accounts transferred to out-of-town agencies may put the fee at a higher percentage.

An agency should not be judged by the percentage of its commission alone. Rate of recovery is an equally important consideration. Just because a group pays less for an agency's services does not mean it is getting a bargain. In fact, the group may be hurting itself financially and endangering its public image by using a less expensive and less effective collection agency. In some cases, it may be advantageous to go with the agency charging the higher rate. The importance of both rate of recovery and commission charged by the agency is illustrated by the agency comparison in *Figure 12-1*.

It is the net return that counts, not the contingency fee. The net recovery after commission is the key financial factor. However, there is also the public relations factor to consider. Extremely rigid collection techniques can increase recovery rate at the expense of a medical group's reputation.

FIGURE 12-1.
COMPARISON OF TWO COLLECTION AGENCIES

COLLECTION AGENCY	AGENCY A	AGENCY B
Total dollars submitted	$25,000	$25,000
Gross amount collected	$15,000	$ 7,000
Percent recovery rate (collections to submissions)	60%	28%
Commissions paid	$ 5,250	$ 1,750
Percent paid (commissions to collections)	35%	25%
Total net recovery	$ 9,750	$ 5,250
Percent net recovery rate*	39%	21%

*Divide total net recovery by total dollars submitted.

All facets of a collection agency's reputation should be considered before one is chosen. The U.S. Department of Commerce Small Business Bulletin No. 472 reads as follows: "Those [collection] agencies whose rates might seem high to you at first glance in many instances will offer a more complete service."

Complaints from former patients who have been referred to an agency may be biased. So, above all, it is important to keep an open mind and get all the facts concerning complaints before taking any action. It is up to the medical group to make certain its agency is using sound judgment in its collection techniques at all times.

Regular Listings and Cancellation of Accounts

Accounts should be listed on a regular basis with the third-party collector. The accounts determined to be forwarded for collection can be set in a follow-up file and listed with the agency at least once a month, on about the same day each month, to avoid added delays in collection efforts.

It is advantageous to place an account with the collector as quickly as possible after it has been decided that the account should be forwarded. Collection agency figures show that the accounts from medical groups who list regularly are more collectible, and a higher percentage of gross and net collection is obtained. Time is crucial in collections.

A medical group has the right to cancel any account which has been placed with an agency. However, lack of collection should not be used as the lone reason for return. It is important to get all the facts first, then pass fair judgment on the account before asking the agency to cancel. The agency must be notified in writing to discontinue all collection activities on the account to be returned. The agency is then allowed a "reasonable period of time" to close its files and return the account to the medical group.

Some agencies may reply to a cancellation request with a statement similar to this: "A judgment has been made on the account and we have turned it over to our attorney to contemplate suing; therefore, we do not feel you should take the account away from us." If an agency responds in this manner, some investigation should be done to determine whether or not any legal action has actually been started. If it has, it is necessary to review the medical group's business arrangement with the agency, study and reevaluate the account in question, and most importantly, use sound judgment in making any decision. If no legal action has been initiated, the agency should be approached again. The objective in this case is to reach a consensus as to the next step to take with the account. It must be kept in mind that the medical group's image is at stake. Public relations extend not only to patients, but also to the businesses with which the group engages.

Evaluation Criteria

So far in this strategy, it has been pointed out that a third party is a necessary tool in medical credit management, and the advantages of this arrangement and agency selection criteria have been discussed. The next step is the evaluation of collection agencies currently servicing accounts.

How much are they collecting? Dividing the amount submitted during the last year, two months prior to the figuring date, into the amount collected to date will give a true picture of the agencies' actual collection abilities. Agencies cannot be expected to collect a high percentage of accounts recently submitted to them, and basing evaluation on these figures would give a misleading percentage of the agencies' ability to collect. Collection percentage will depend somewhat on the aging of the account when it is turned over, the amount of work put into the account by the group before it is turned over, group policy in governing collection activity, and other factors.

What are they charging? The next step is to determine what the agency is charging the medical group. Dividing the total amount submitted into the total amount of collection agency fee over the same period (or dividing the total submitted into the group's net collection and subtracting that figure from 100 percent) will provide the percentage that the agency is charging. It is the net collection that counts.

If recovery percentages from the agency are not satisfactory, it may be necessary to audit the collection activity on bad debt accounts placed with the agency. Even if collection results are satisfactory, an audit will assure that the agency's collection practices and dunning notices are consistent with the message the medical group wants to portray to patients. The following tips offer advice on how to handle and what to look for in an agency audit:

1.   First, bring a list of accounts to be audited. Do not let the agency "prepare" the accounts. The list should include a mixture of paid accounts, accounts

closed and returned as uncollectible, active accounts, and legal accounts, if applicable.

2. Review all dunning notices and collection policies to ensure they are consistent with the message the medical group wants to portray to patients.

3. Note how long after placement the agency begins collection activity. A dunning notice should be sent to the patient within days after the account is listed, and followed up by a telephone contact within one week.

4. If the patient has not been contacted, review the length of time between attempts. Is the agency utilizing late nights or Saturdays for contact attempts?

5. Review all accounts which were closed and returned as uncollectible for sufficient collection activity. Was the patient given enough opportunity to pay? Did the agency complete adequate skiptracing steps if it was unable to locate the debtor?

6. Review the paid accounts to see what type of activity was taken to get payment. This can reveal a great deal about the medical group collection department. If the agency receives a good portion of its payments simply by resubmitting a claim to a third-party carrier, it is imperative to take a look at the group's own billing and collection areas.

7. On legal accounts, make certain the patient had sufficient opportunity to pay voluntarily. Unnecessary legal action can be costly for the medical group and can harm public relations.

8. Sit and observe a collector while visiting the agency. Obviously, the collector hosting the visit will be on best behavior, so a good trick is to listen to the other collectors while appearing to observe just one.

9. Watch for small monthly payment plans without supporting financial documentation. All efforts for payment in full should be exhausted (credit card, bank financing, etc.), before setting up the patient with small payment arrangements. If a payment plan has been set, be sure the agency follows up with the patient every few months to see if the debtor's financial situation has changed at all.

Although the collection agency is a separate organization, patients still view it as an extension of the medical group. While its tactics must be more aggressive than those of the medical group, the agency's actions should be consistent with maintaining favorable patient relations. The following are further considerations:

•   Do not hesitate to have a particular collector removed from working the medical group's business if numerous complaints on the collection approach are received.

•   Medical group staff should not be spending excessive time copying or researching information on agency accounts. Most agencies will supply one of their employees to come to the medical group facility to do the work.

- A maximum time limit (six months) can be set for collection efforts. At that time, the account should be closed at the first agency and placed with a second. This gives the first agency an incentive to collect quickly. In addition, the second agency has the incentive to do well hoping to win over first placements.

Investigating Other Agencies

After exploring what is wanted in an agency and what the current agency is doing, it is important to find out if someone else can do a better job. This can be accomplished through an investigation of other agencies. A list of clients should be obtained from prospective agencies, and the clients called to determine the quality of the job being done. The standard evaluation questions previously mentioned can be discussed, as well as prompt remittance, public relations, accurate reporting, and other areas of concern. Most companies keep records with this same type of information.

Another approach is to contact other medical groups, hospitals, and doctors' offices in the area. Is there one agency that has more medical clients than others? If so, there must be a good reason for it.

A written report of the investigation should be kept so that figures can be compared when the survey has been completed. If there are one or two agencies whose work seems to stand out from the others, it may prove to be worth the effort to go one step further with them. A personal call to their offices will provide an opportunity to see what kind of collectors are actually doing the calling and to listen to them collect. Are they desirable individuals for working the medical group accounts? Form letters can also be reviewed, as well as the exact procedures that will be followed on accounts. Close attention should be paid to the order and cleanliness of the office. If the overall impression is that an agency other than the one currently being used can be more effective, it may be time for a change.

Attorneys for Collection

Who gets better collection results — collection agencies or attorneys? If volume only is judged, the answer is collection agencies. However, some medical groups are using attorneys for collection services. Assuming contingency fees for collection activity are competitively priced, there are some definite benefits to this approach:

- Impact on patients when a letter is received from an attorney
- Patient perspective that this matter is more serious and a legal suit is eminent
- Attorney ability to file suit quicker and for less cost
- Attorney ability to spread legal costs over numerous accounts
- Ability of attorney to deal with other attorneys in accident cases

Most collection agencies offer legal services, too, so all options should be explored. However, the collection agent who provides the best net return is the one to use.

Importance of Analysis

Is all this really necessary? Can any improvement really come of this? Aren't all agencies similar in method and results?   They are not, and the manager's responsibility to the medical group, the community, and himself or herself is to find out if the best possible collection results are being obtained, both financially and in patient relations. Good results mean a savings in dollars, and the all-important factor of public relations can improve as well.

It is well worth the time and trouble to: (1) determine the value of third-party collection to a particular situation, (2) evaluate the type of work now being done for the group, and (3) investigate other agencies and the merits of changing agencies for a more profitable collection operation. The choice of any agency can make a sizeable difference in the overall collection results obtained and the quality of service performed for the medical group.

Keeping close tabs of the accounts turned over for collection is usually an undesirable task and often not done at all. However, being aware of the percentage collected by agencies can help in determining the quality of the job being done, and may be helpful when a change is being considered. An agency analysis report form is provided in *Worksheet 16* in Appendix A.

Considering an In-House Agency

The use of collection agencies is normally an important link in the chain of a strong collection program. Depending on the size of a medical group and its collection staff, agencies may be relied on to play an active role in increasing total cash flow. Traditionally, group practices have utilized outside professional collection agencies; however, an in-house system is a viable alternative.

Today, many medical group administrators are considering establishing an in-house collection agency. Under the right conditions, an in-house agency helps to contain costs by eliminating the medical group's outside collection agency expenses. Efficient in-house collection often speeds up cash turnaround. However, all aspects of a system must be considered before an in-house agency can be set up.

The first step in developing an in-house collection agency is discussion with and investigation by the medical group's attorneys. They can determine the legal ramifications for the group and the community, and they will outline procedures for setting up the agency's necessary qualifications. Since this may vary by state and approach, it is important to clear this hurdle before time is spent planning the project. If there are no serious legal obstacles, the advantages and disadvantages of an in-house collection agency may then be determined.

Some advantages are pertinent only to a particular medical group, but several are generally applicable. An in-house agency can give greater internal control over the accounts written off and the actual collection of accounts previously referred to an agency. Since agency staff members are selected, there is direct control over the personnel who represent the group in collection and processing of accounts. As such, an in-house collection agency may intensify a group's public relations efforts.

With staff trained in the collection philosophy of the institution, the entire collection process reflects the medical group's image.

The real payoff for the medical group can be reduced collection expense and improved cash flow. Analysis shows that medical groups of more than 30 physicians, with a write-off in excess of 3 percent of gross revenue to third-party collections, should be able to substantially reduce their collection expenses by developing an in-house agency to collect their otherwise referred accounts. Because an in-house agency initiates third-party collection procedures at an earlier stage and generally has more ability to concentrate efforts on specific cases, this arrangement may speed turnaround time and strengthen a group practice's cash flow.

On the other hand, an in-house collection agency may cost more than the agency currently being used. The medical group may lack experience in developing, implementing, and operating an organization of this nature. Running a medical group business office is very different from operating a collection agency. Often, in-house agencies fail because the medical group lacks knowledge of bad debt collection methods, personnel requirements, and the profit- oriented thinking necessary for success. Minor disadvantages to consider include the initial funding expense and the cold fact that a qualified collection manager and good collectors are difficult to locate in many areas of the country.

If after weighing the advantages and disadvantages of developing an in-house collection agency, there seems to be no doubt that such a unit would be beneficial to the medical group, the possible savings in collection expenses must be determined. The first step is to estimate the dollar amount generally referred to an agency within a year and to project the recovery. Next, the approximate gross operating expense for the initial year of an in-house agency should be compared to the projected recovery figure. This determines the profit or loss for the year. Then, this figure can be contrasted with the expense of the present system.

Computation of this profit or loss margin for a two-year to three-year period will help to provide a clear picture of the potential savings over a longer period of time. If the ratio of expense to profit is considered, as well as recovery figures for the group-controlled agency compared to that of commercial agencies, the first year is often a break-even year. However, usually by the end of the second year of operation, the group-controlled agency's recovery rate increases. Collection expenses decrease and sizable profits are realized. Consequently, cash flow is improved at a lower cost level to the medical group.

The accuracy of projected operating expenses is directly related to the ability to estimate profits gained in the development of an in-house collection unit. To determine operating expenses, an accurate projection should be made of the number of accounts referred in a year. Staffing requirements, postage, telephone services, printing expenses, legal fees, and data processing needs are dependent upon account volume. Because the agency should be in a location removed from the medical group, another major expense is rent.

Staff expense will constitute the largest expense. Knowledge of staffing requirements for an in-house agency is critical to its financial success. Overstaffing will inflate expenses and reduce profits. Understaffing will reduce collection totals due to many factors. Overburdened staff members become unmotivated and generally have little time for public relations amenities, or time to devote attention to or make sufficient contacts with the persons involved.

A general rule of thumb is that one collector can effectively handle 2,000 to 2,500 accounts at any given time. Of course, this varies with the collector's experience and skill. Another general rule calls for 1.4 full-time-equivalent (FTE) clerical positions for every 2,000 new accounts listed each month. There are variables in clerical needs. The number of new accounts to set up, work cards to prepare, amount of filing, acknowledgments, purging, refiling, follow-ups, among other concerns, should be considered. The quantity of incoming and outgoing mail and correspondence to be typed or processed must also be determined.

Salary projections are dependent on the manner in which collectors and clerical personnel are paid. Their salaries can be determined by base plus commission or total commission. Clerical personnel are generally paid by the hour, on a weekly or monthly basis.

Since the telephone is a major expense item, the number of outgoing telephone calls per collector and the potential expense of a WATS line must be considered. A gauge of 60 to 70 telephone calls per day per collector can be used for determining telephone expenses.

If a definite savings in collection expenses can be forecast and other advantages for developing an in-house collection agency can be suggested that are pertinent to a group's long-range plans, only then is it appropriate to present the idea to the medical group's governing body. A well-prepared document should include all rationale previously discussed as well as unique selling points. It is important to remember to account for an organization's distinctive needs when planning a presentation of an in-house collection unit. Total commitment is essential before going to the medical group governing body with the idea.

Going into Action

After board approval, the plan for a group-controlled agency should be discussed with state and local government officials to be sure the proposal meets specific regulations for a licensed collection agency. An application for license may have to be sent to the state commissioner's office for approval prior to qualifying for an agency license. The name of the agency should be included, as well as proof of bonding requirements, floor plan, financial statement, corporation articles and bylaws, and layout of any forms to be used in collection attempts. The state commissioner's office may require an annual audit, an annual financial statement or annual report, and an annual license renewal. Liability insurance is also necessary for protection against any legal action which may be taken against the agency.

One key to the success of an in-house agency will be the image or identity that is portrayed to the public. The collection agency must appear to be independent of the medical group management. The agency's effectiveness will be hurt if it appears to the patient as controlled by the practice. Being identified as a division of the office negates one key advantage of a collection agency. Specifically, if the agency is perceived as an independent company, it is not restricted by the same public relations limitations as the medical group. If an in-house agency does not have a separate and distinct identity and is not portrayed as a collection agency, it will be no more effective than the business office.

Opening to Other Clients

Before the services of an in-house agency are offered to other medical clients to generate additional revenue for the medical group, the following points should be considered:

- Most importantly, do not offer services at a reduced commission rate; this tactic will eventually eat into profits. Charge the going commission rate in the area and do not discount the commission for referral volume. Clients with a higher commission rate, such as physicians, increase the profit margin.

- Spread out the client base. Do not become tied to just a few major clients. Should they decide to reduce or eliminate their referrals, the in-house agency could suddenly be overstaffed, and the profit margin would decline immediately.

- Carefully analyze recovery totals and percentages by client and collector. This determines the most profitable and unprofitable clients and the most productive and unproductive collectors.

- Sell the group's collection services with attractive promotional brochures and advertisements. Services such as precollection notices, educational workshops, and accounts receivable consulting may also be offered. In any case, a good marketing plan is important to the success of any commercial agency in the open marketplace.

An Answer, A Challenge, and a Risk

As a particular situation is analyzed, it may be discovered that an in-house collection agency is an effective answer to many medical group financial and account control problems. An in-house agency may:

- Reduce collection expense
- Improve cash flow
- Give more direct control on status of accounts
- Allow firsthand management of collection techniques
- Increase personal supervision of collection staff
- Unify collection philosophy within the medical group

An in-house collection agency adds a new and challenging dimension to the manager's job. At the same time, there are risks involved. It is important not to overlook any potential operating expense items, including the following:

- Manager's salary (including commission)
- Clerks' salaries
- Collectors' salaries, and commissions
- Employees' fringe benefits packages
- Rental of office space
- Postage and post office box rental
- Printing (notices, envelopes)
- Office supplies
- Equipment (desks, chairs, typewriters, adding machines)
- Data processing computer
- Travel expenses for additional education of staff
- Liability insurance, bonding costs, and license fees
- Attorney fees
- Telephone services

Projections for the first year of operation for an in-house collection agency should be based on estimates from previous years' data from out-of-house collection agencies. Both the best and worst scenarios should be considered in order to develop a thorough understanding of the initial set-up costs. A form for projecting first-year costs of operation of an in-house collection agency is provided in Worksheet 17 in Appendix A.

If after all the analyses, projections, and considerations have been made, the decision is made to develop an in-house collection agency, the key to success is a strong commitment at the outset. Steps to setting up an in-house agency are provided in *Figure 12-2*.

FIGURE 12-2.
STEPS TO SETTING UP AN IN-HOUSE COLLECTION AGENCY

1. Obtain legal opinion.

2. Determine feasibility and timetable for implementation.

3. Present proposal to board of directors or governing body for approval.

4. Obtain license (if necessary).

5. Develop procedures, policies, and data processing report formats.

6. Design collection notices and letters.

7. Obtain office space and equipment.

8. Hire and train staff.

**SUMMARY OF
KEY STRATEGY 12**

As a collection strategy is developed for past due accounts, consider the following:

1. Any outside collection agency utilized should be considered an extension of the collection department. Open communications are essential.

2. An outside agency should be chosen carefully, after thorough investigation. An agency should be selected based on its merits.

3. Any outside agency chosen should have a public relations policy that is compatible with the medical group's philosophy.

4. Monitoring and auditing collection agency activities may be helpful in obtaining better results. Periodic evaluations should be part of the agreement with the agency.

5. If cost effectiveness is a concern, total net recovery after the agency's commissions have been paid really counts.

6. Overseeing write-offs to agencies is an essential part of an efficient total cash flow program.

7. If outside collection agency costs are stifling medical group cash flow, setting up an in-house agency may solve the problem.

8. Setting up an in-house collection agency should be considered only after a close examination of medical group expenses and projected recovery indicates that it would be more profitable for the group, or it is felt that the medical group staff would thus be able to do a much better public relations job.

9. Some advantages of an in-house agency include more direct control of overdue accounts, a unified collection philosophy, and increased supervision of the collection staff.

10. Disadvantages of an in-house agency are the cost of establishing such a system and finding qualified personnel to run it.

APPENDIX A: WORKSHEETS

1. Daily Billing Control Sheet

2. Monthly Billing Control Report

3. Weekly Unbilled Insurance Report

4. Third-Party Profile

5. Third-Party Analysis Fact Sheet

6. Self-Pay Debtor Profile

7. Accounts Receivable Analysis Worksheet

8. Pinpointing Key Result Areas

9. Key Result Areas and Performance Indicators

10. Monthly Goal Status Report

11. Annual Action Plan

12. Comparative Analysis of Actual to Projected Goal

13. Formula to Reach Goal

14. Collector's Monthly Status Report

15. Accounts Receivable Status Report

16. Agency Analysis Report

17. Projected First Year of Operation for an In-House Collection Agency

NOTE: The worksheet documents contained in this appendix may be reproduced, provided the copyright notation on each worksheet appears on each reproduction.

WORKSHEET 1
DAILY BILLING CONTROL SHEET

Prepared by ______________________________   Date ____________________

Financial Class	Received		Billed		Backlog	
	Number	**Amount**	**Number**	**Amount**	**Number**	**Amount**
Blue Cross/ Blue Shield	_______	_______	_______	_______	_______	_______
Medicare	_______	_______	_______	_______	_______	_______
Medicaid	_______	_______	_______	_______	_______	_______
Third Party	_______	_______	_______	_______	_______	_______
Self-Pay	_______	_______	_______	_______	_______	_______
Other	_______	_______	_______	_______	_______	_______
Totals	_______	_______	_______	_______	_______	_______

WORKSHEET 2
MONTHLY BILLING CONTROL REPORT

Prepared by ______________________________________   Date ____________________

Assignment Distribution

Biller	Blue Cross/ Blue Shield Number/Amt.	Medicare Number/Amt.	Medicaid Number/Amt.	Third Party Number/Amt.	Self-Pay Number/Amt.
A	__________	__________	__________	__________	__________
B	__________	__________	__________	__________	__________
C	__________	__________	__________	__________	__________
D	__________	__________	__________	__________	__________
E	__________	__________	__________	__________	__________
Totals	__________	__________	__________	__________	__________

Actual Billings

Biller	Blue Cross/ Blue Shield Number/Amt.	Medicare Number/Amt.	Medicaid Number/Amt.	Third Party Number/Amt.	Self-Pay Number/Amt.
A	__________	__________	__________	__________	__________
B	__________	__________	__________	__________	__________
C	__________	__________	__________	__________	__________
D	__________	__________	__________	__________	__________
E	__________	__________	__________	__________	__________
Totals	__________	__________	__________	__________	__________

WORKSHEET 3
WEEKLY UNBILLED INSURANCE REPORT

Prepared by ___________________________________   Date _______________________

| | **Current Week** | | **Previous Week** | |
	Number	Amount	Number	Amount
Carry over from previous week ·	_________	_________	_________	_________
Charges incurred during current week	_________	_________	_________	_________
Total available for processing	_________	_________	_________	_________
Billings processed and mailed	_________	_________	_________	_________
Total unbilled insurance	_________	_________	_________	_________

Breakdown of Claims Processed

	Number	Amount	Number	Amount
Blue Cross/Blue Shield	_________	_________	_________	_________
Medicare	_________	_________	_________	_________
Medicaid	_________	_________	_________	_________
Third Party	_________	_________	_________	_________
Other	_________	_________	_________	_________
Total unbilled insurance (same as above)	_________	_________	_________	_________

WORKSHEET 4
THIRD-PARTY PROFILE

Prepared by ____ Date ________________

Third Party Name	Number of Days since Billing	Position of Contacted Person	Approx. Time on Job	Reasons for Nonpayment in Past or within Next 48 Hours
_____________	_______	_________	________	__________________________
_____________	_______	_________	________	__________________________
_____________	_______	_________	________	__________________________
_____________	_______	_________	________	__________________________
_____________	_______	_________	________	__________________________
_____________	_______	_________	________	__________________________
_____________	_______	_________	________	__________________________

SUMMARY:

A. Five Most Commonly Dealt With Insurance Companies:

  1. ____
  2. ____
  3. ____
  4. ____
  5. ____

B. Average Number of Days since Billing:

  ____

C. Two Most Common Positions of Personnel Contacted about Accounts:

  1. ____
  2. ____

D. Average Approximate Time at That Position:

  ____

E. Five Major Reasons Given for Nonpayment:

  1. ____
  2. ____
  3. ____
  4. ____
  5. ____

WORKSHEET 5
THIRD-PARTY ANALYSIS FACT SHEET

____

Prepared by ____   Date ___________________

____

Third Party Company ____

Local Address ____

Home Office ____

Annual Account Volume $ _____________________ (How much do we bill them annually?)

Average Turnaround Time (from billing to payment) _______________ As of ______

Average Number of Phone Contacts on Delinquent Accounts ___________________

____

	Name	Overall Experience	Experience with This Company	Reports to
1. Claims Manager	_____	_____	_____	_____
2. Claims Supervisor	_____	_____	_____	_____
3. Processing Clerk	_____	_____	_____	_____

Most Contacts with ____

Process for Payment at Above Address ______ Yes   ______ No

If Not — Where Do Claims Go for Payment? _______________________________

Name and Title of Contact Person _______________________________________

Address ___________________________   Phone _______________________

Sequence of Steps for Processing Claims for Payment at this Organization:

1. _____________________________   4. _____________________________

2. _____________________________   5. _____________________________

3. _____________________________   6. _____________________________

Major Reasons for Delay or Nonpayment of Claims:

1. ____

2. ____

3. ____

4. ____

Steps that Can be Taken to Speed Up Payment of Claims:

1. ____

2. ____

3. ____

4. ____

Remarks: ____

WORKSHEET 6
SELF-PAY DEBTOR PROFILE

Prepared by ____   Date _____________________

Age of Debtor	Blue Collar or White Collar	Zip Code	Time on Job	Reasons for Nonpayment
_____	_________	_________	_________	_____________________________
_____	_________	_________	_________	_____________________________
_____	_________	_________	_________	_____________________________
_____	_________	_________	_________	_____________________________
_____	_________	_________	_________	_____________________________
_____	_________	_________	_________	_____________________________
_____	_________	_________	_________	_____________________________
_____	_________	_________	_________	_____________________________
_____	_________	_________	_________	_____________________________
_____	_________	_________	_________	_____________________________
_____	_________	_________	_________	_____________________________
_____	_________	_________	_________	_____________________________
_____	_________	_________	_________	_____________________________
_____	_________	_________	_________	_____________________________
_____	_________	_________	_________	_____________________________
_____	_________	_________	_________	_____________________________
_____	_________	_________	_________	_____________________________
_____	_________	_________	_________	_____________________________

SUMMARY:

A. Average Age of Debtor: _____________

B. Percent of White Collar: _____________

C. Percent of Blue Collar: _____________

D. Most Common Zip Code: _____________

E. Average Time on Job: _____________

F. Five Major Reasons Given for Nonpayment:
1. _________________________________
2. _________________________________
3. _________________________________
4. _________________________________
5. _________________________________

WORKSHEET 7
ACCOUNTS RECEIVABLE ANALYSIS WORKSHEET

Prepared by _________________________   Date _________________

Accounts Receivable Category	Step-by-Step Performance Procedures	Responsibilities Delegated	To Whom/ Position	Analytical Reports Needed

WORKSHEET 8
PINPOINTING KEY RESULT AREAS

Prepared by _____________________________________   Date ____________________

Most Important Areas within My Responsibility	Percentage Level of Importance*
1. ____	__________
2. ____	__________
3. ____	__________
4. ____	__________
5. ____	__________
6. ____	__________
7. ____	__________
8. ____	__________
9. ____	__________
10. ____	__________
11. ____	__________
	100%

*Assign a percentage to each area in terms of its importance to your total area of responsibility, so that the cumulative figure does not exceed 100%.

WORKSHEET 9
KEY RESULT AREAS AND PERFORMANCE INDICATORS

Prepared by _________________________________   Date _______________

Key Result Area Level of Importance	Performance Indicator	Acceptable Result	Expected Result	Possible Result

WORKSHEET 10
MONTHLY GOAL STATUS REPORT

Prepared by ____   Date ____________________

Period ____

Key Result Area Level of Importance	Performance Indicator	Acceptable Result	Expected Result	Possible Result	Status at Month End

WORKSHEET 11
ANNUAL ACTION PLAN

Prepared by ___________________________________   Date ____________________

Period ____

Key Result Area	Goal	Projections		Actual	
		Action Planned	Commencing Date - Completion Date	Date Action Taken	Comments: Including Reasons for Action Not Taken or Changes in Plan

WORKSHEET 12
COMPARATIVE ANALYSIS OF ACTUAL TO PROJECTED GOAL

Prepared by _________________________________ Date _________________

Collection Category	Actual		Goal		
	Outstanding Months AR	Outstanding Amount	Outstanding Months AR	Outstanding Amount	Amount to Reduce
Self-Pay	_______	_______	_______	_______	_______
Third Party	_______	_______	_______	_______	_______
Medicare	_______	_______	_______	_______	_______
Medicaid	_______	_______	_______	_______	_______
Blue Cross/ Blue Shield	_______	_______	_______	_______	_______
Other	_______	_______	_______	_______	_______
Total		_______		_______	_______

WORKSHEET 13
FORMULA TO REACH GOAL

Prepared by _______________________________   Date _______________

Collection Category	Actual		Goal	
	Amount to Reduce	Average Billings per Week	Average Collection Goal per Week	Gain per Month
Self-Pay	_________	_________	_________	_________
Third Party	_________	_________	_________	_________
Medicare	_________	_________	_________	_________
Medicaid	_________	_________	_________	_________
Blue Cross/ Blue Shield	_________	_________	_________	_________
Other	_________	_________	_________	_________
Total	_________	_________	_________	_________

Ideas to improve plan and reach goals: _______________________________

____

____

____

WORKSHEET 14
COLLECTOR'S MONTHLY STATUS REPORT

Name of Collector ____

Prepared by _________________________________ Date _______________

Month of ____

____

Distribution:
Administrator ____
Business manager ____
Billing supervisor ____
Collection manager ____

	Actual Collections	Goal
Week #1	_________________	_________________
Week #2	_________________	_________________
Week #3	_________________	_________________
Week #4	_________________	_________________
Average for month	_________________	_________________
Average for last month	_________________	_________________
Average for year-to-date	_________________	_________________

WORKSHEET 15
ACCOUNTS RECEIVABLE STATUS REPORT

Prepared by _______________________________   Date _______________

Collection Category	Actual			Goal	
	Outstanding Amount	Outstanding Months A/R	Amount over 60 days	Outstanding Months A/R	Outstanding Amount
Self-Pay	_______	_______	_______	_______	_______
Third Party	_______	_______	_______	_______	_______
Medicare	_______	_______	_______	_______	_______
Medicaid	_______	_______	_______	_______	_______
Blue Cross/ Blue Shield	_______	_______	_______	_______	_______
Other	_______	_______	_______	_______	_______
Total	_______		_______		_______

WORKSHEET 16
AGENCY ANALYSIS REPORT

Prepared by _________________________________   Date _______________

<u>Collection Agencies</u>	<u>Agency A</u>	<u>Agency B</u>
Total Dollars Submitted YTD	_____________	_____________
This Month's Collection	_____________	_____________
Gross Amount Collected to Date	_____________	_____________
Total Percentage of Gross Collections	_____________	_____________
Commissions Paid	_____________	_____________
Percent of Commissions to Collections	_____________	_____________
Percent of Net Collection to Total Submitted*	_____________	_____________

*Subtract commissions paid total from gross collections and divide by total submitted for net recovery percentage.

WORKSHEET 17
PROJECTED FIRST YEAR OF OPERATION FOR AN IN-HOUSE COLLECTION AGENCY

Prepared by ______________________   Date ______________________

Item	Jan	Feb	Mar	Apr	May	Jun	Jul	Aug	Sep	Oct	Nov	Dec	Total
Number of Accounts Listed													
Amount Listed													
Projected Collections													
Percent of Gross Outstanding Balance to Amount Listed													
Gross Operating Expense													
Projected Profit or Loss													

NOTE: Use estimated figures based on previous years' data from out-of-house collection agencies. Complete this form for both the best and worst scenarios in order to develop a thorough understanding of the initial costs of setting up an in-house collection agency.

BIBLIOGRAPHY

American Collectors Association. *A Manual on the Fair Debt Collection Practices Act.* Minneapolis: American Collectors Association, Inc., 1979.

American Medical Association. *Current Procedural Terminology.* 4th ed. Chicago: American Medical Association, 1992.

Anderson, S. T.   "Dealing With Reimbursement Difficulties in Today's Payment Environment." *Medical Group Management Journal* 38 no. 3 (1991): 44-49.

Appleby, C. R. "Out of the Abyss." *HealthWeek* 3 no. 17 (1989): 18-20.

Aquino, F. "Decisive Dealings With Collection Agencies." *Medical Group Management* 33 no. 6 (1986): 46.

Berry, M. J. "Analyze Your Practice's Collection Management System." *American Medical News* 33 no. 38 (1990): 15.

Brooks, L. B. "Improving Cash Flow — Electronic Claims Processing." *College Review* 6 no. 2 (Fall 1989): 58-64.

Clarkin, J. F.   "Back Office Functions of the Billing Process." *Topics in Health Care Financing* 17 no. 1 (1990): 39-66.

"Collecting Your Fees From Divorced or Separated Patients." *The Physician's Advisory* 85 no. 3 (1985): 10.

Comeau, J. F. "Collections Systems That Deter Lawsuits." *Physician's Management* 32 no. 2 (1992): 113-118.

Crane, M. "Let Patients Pay You With Plastic?" *Medical Economics* 68 no. 12 (1991): 117-122.

Dingess, B. "Collecting More from Insurance Companies." *Journal of Patient Account Management* 12 no. 6 (1983): 6.

Elder, D. L. "Accounts Receivable Management Techniques." *Medical Group Management* 32 no. 4 (1985): 30.

Elder, D. L. "Collection Time Again." *Medical Group Management* 31 no. 6 (1984): 20.

Fox, Y. M. "8 Crucial Steps to Successful Collections." *Physician's Management* 31 no. 7 (July 1991): 88.

Gareiss, R. "A Reluctance to Charge Ahead." *American Medical News* 33 no. 34 (1990): 13.

Gray, J. "Games Insurers Play With Your Reimbursements." *Medical Economics* 67 no. 18 (1990): 162.

Harrison, R. L. "Anatomy of a Collection System." *Medical Group Management* 27 no. 6 (1980): 54.

"Helpful Abbreviations for Recording Delinquent Collection Phone Calls." *The Physician's Advisory* 88 no. 10 (1988): 6.

Henderson, T. M. "Getting the Most From Your Private Pay Accounts." *Medical Group Management* 33 no. 1 (1986): 42.

Herrin, D., comp. *Directory of Software Vendors for Group Practice 1992*. Englewood: Medical Group Management Association, 1992.

"'Hire-Up' for a Reimbursement Expert; You Need a Good Person for Billing and Insurance Coding." *The Physician's Advisory* 90 no. 7 (1990): 1-2.

Hogan, C. "Pre-Admitting and Receivables." *Journal of Patient Accounts Management* 15 no. 3: 7.

"How to Appeal Your Disappointing Insurance Payments." *The Physician's Advisory* 91 no. 7 (1991): 5-6.

"How to Calculate Certain Basic Management Ratios." *The Physician's Advisory* 85 no. 3 (1985): 6.

"How to Reduce Carrier Payment Denials." *The Internist* 32 no. 6 (1991): 37.

"How to Select Your Collection Agency." *The Physician's Advisory* 89 no. 9 (1989): 6.

"How to Track Your 'In-Office' Collections." *The Physician's Advisory* 89 no. 8 (1989): 1-2.

"How Well Should Your Collection Agency Perform?" *The Physician's Advisory* 90 no. 2 (1990): 7.

Johnston, L. J., and Barazsu, P. J. "Making Automated Billing Stronger." *Medical Group Management* 33 no. 2 (1986): 30-33.

Kadas, R. M., and Butler. T. J. "The '90s Paradigm Shift for Electronic Claims." *Computers in Healthcare* 13 no. 1 (1992): 46-48.

Kanter, R.M. *The Change Masters: Innovation for Productivity in the American Corporation*. New York: Simon and Schuster, 1983.

"Key Steps to Improving Billing and Collections Procedures." *Physicians Financial News* 7 no. 8 (1989): P4.

Koenig, D. "What No Collection Agency Can Ever Do for You." *Medical Economics* 68 no. 13 (1991): 82.

Kurt, E. J., Jr. "Collection Tactics That Can Get You Sued." *Medical Economics* 67 no. 6 (1990): 119.

Larkin, H. "Electronic Filing Brings Billing Boon." *American Medical News* 33 no. 36 (1990): 11.

Mann, L. "Credit Cards: A Convenient, Cost-Effective Payment Alternative for Medical Practices." *The Journal of Medical Practice Management* 7 no. 1 (1991): 24-28.

Mann, L. "Credit Cards: The Practical Payment Alternative." *Group Practice Journal* 40 no. 6 (1991): 56-58.

Mathe, N. "Electronic Claims Speed Medicare Payments." *Ophthalmology Management* 9 no. 4 (1991): 28.

McKenney, P. C. "How to Get Paid on the Spot." *Physician's Management* 32 no. 1 (1992): 113.

Miller, C. S., and Wolpoff, H. K. "The Internal Woe of the Physician's Office." *Medical Group Management Journal* 38 no. 6 (1991): 57.

Monaco, C. "Electronic Media Claims: Savings Cited by Users." *Part B News* 5 no. 20 (1991): 8-12.

Mowll, C. A. "Knowing How and When to Grant Credit." *Healthcare Financial Management* 43 no. 2 (1989): 88.

Moynihan, J. J., et al. "Standards Opening a Door to Electronic Payments." *Healthcare Financial Management* 45 no. 3 (1991): 21.

Murray, D. "How to Find—and Use—a Good Collection Agency." *Medical Economics* 67 no. 18 (1990): 83.

Nystrom, D. A., FACMGA. *Compensating for Uncompensated Care.* Englewood: American College of Medical Group Administrators, 1990.

Palmer, D. M., and Palmer, S. H. *The Telephone Handbook for Medical and Dental Practices. Words, Statements, Techniques, and Procedures to Ensure Professional Telephone Communications.* Homewood: Palmer Associates, 1989.

"Payment Books Push Healthcare Expenses Higher on Patient's Priority List." *Physician's Marketing & Management* 4 no. 7 (1991): 1-4.

Pear, M. J. "How Credit Cards Can Improve Cash Flow." *Medical Group Management Journal* 38 no. 6 (1991): 40.

Peters, T.J. and Waterman, Jr., R.H. *In Search of Excellence: Lessons from America's Best-Run Companies*. New York: Harper and Row, 1982.

Peterson, D. "Using an RFP for Collection Agencies." *Patient Accounts* 11 no. 6 (1988): 2-3.

"Plastic is One Answer to Collection Woes for Medical Practices." *Medical Office Manager* 5 no. 12 (1991): 14-15.

Politzer, B. "Claims of Excellence." *HMO Magazine* 32 no. 6 (1991): 38.

Regan, D. M. "Strategies for Receiving Proper Third Party Reimbursement." *Medical Group Management Journal* 36 no. 6 (1989): 36.

Reinke, T. W. "Going With Electronic Financial Management." *Medical Group Management Journal* 36 no. 1 (1989): 26.

Rice, E. W. "Boost Collections Without Losing Patients." *Physician's Management* 29 no. 1 (1989): 66.

Salmon, P. M., and Smith, P. C. "The Most Common Reasons Medicare Rejects Claims." *Physician's Management* 31 no. 2 (1991): 44.

"Set Up Systems to Facilitate Payments After Review of Dealings With Insurers." *Physicians Financial News* 7 no. 8 (1989): P5.

Shaw, P. W. "Appealing Medicare Payment Denials." *Medical Group Management Journal* 38 no. 6 (1991): 26.

Skeesick, G. "Coping With Managed Care in the Business Office." *Patient Accounts* 14 no. 4 (1991): 3.

Slater, R. M., et al. "Giving Receivables an 'Outside' Chance." *Healthcare Financial Management* 45 no. 10 (1991): 56.

"Small Balances Create Big Collection Problems." *Patient Accounts* 12 no. 3: 4.

Solomon, R. J. "Getting a Grip On Collections That Have Gone Out of Control." *American Medical News* 35 no. 7 (1992): 22.

Strahan, H. "A Wise Choice for Your Practice." *Computers in Healthcare* 13 no. 2 (1992): 51.

Sugarman, M. D. "Analyze Your Collections Before Changing Your Policies." *Physicians Financial News* 8 no. 8 (1990): P6.

Sullivan, M. *Development of a Billing and Collections System for a New Joint Venture.* Englewood: American College of Medical Group Administrators, 1991.

Sullivan, T. "Medical Practice Trends: Payers Turning to Practice Audits to Contain Costs and Identify Claims Abuse." *The Journal of Medical Practice Management* 7 no. 1 (1991): 31-35.

Thomas, M. C. "What if Your Patient's Insurance is Bogus?" *Medical Economics* 68 no. 4 (1991): 36-40.

"Using Credit Cards? Emphasize Convenience." *On Managing. . .* 2 no. 2 (1992): 2.

Weinstein, E. S. "Doctors Should Proceed Cautiously When Hiring Collection Agencies." *Physicians Financial News* 7 no. 2 (1989): 27.

"Why Collecting by Credit Card is Worth the Cost." *The Physician's Advisory* 91 no. 1 (1991): 7.

"Your Third Party Insurance I.Q." *The Physician's Advisory* 89 no. 7 (1989): 2-3.

Zupko, K. A. "Easy Ways to Get Paid Faster." *Medical Economics* 67 no. 13 (1990): 61.